STAYING ALIVE
IN TOXIC TIMES

In Memoriam
Dr David Freed

STAYING ALIVE
IN TOXIC TIMES

A Seasonal Guide to Lifelong Health

Dr Jenny Goodman

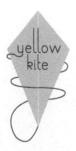

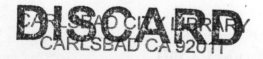

First published in Great Britain in 2020 by Yellow Kite
An imprint of Hodder & Stoughton
An Hachette UK company

3

A CIP catalogue record for this title is available from the British Library

Hardback ISBN 978 1 529 30681 1
eBook ISBN 978 1 529 30830 3

Typeset in Celeste by
Palimpsest Book Production Ltd, Falkirk, Stirlingshire

Printed and bound in Great Britain by Clays Ltd, Elcograf S.p.A.

Hodder & Stoughton policy is to use papers that are natural, renewable and recyclable products and made from wood grown in sustainable forests. The logging and manufacturing processes are expected to conform to the environmental regulations of the country of origin.

Yellow Kite
Hodder & Stoughton Ltd
Carmelite House
50 Victoria Embankment
London EC4Y 0DZ

www.yellowkitebooks.co.uk

CONTENTS

INTRODUCTION

In this book I will show you how you can become seriously healthy, alert and energetic. The need is urgent; many people are feeling needlessly under the weather, or so tired and foggy-brained that they can't even remember what good health feels like. But feeling rubbish is not natural or normal or inevitable. There are reasons for it, and there are plenty of simple, effective things we can do to change it. Even though we are all different, there are some principles that apply to all of us, both for becoming well and for staying well. I will explain those principles, and will also show you how to adapt your eating and your living so that it works best for your particular body, at your particular stage of life.

Why I Had To Write This Book

Let me introduce myself. I entered medical school in 1976, an idealistic young woman with three burning questions in my mind:

1 What causes illness?
2 How can we prevent illness?
3 How do we heal the sick?

When I qualified in 1982, I had learnt nothing about questions 1 and 2, and remarkably little about question 3. On the wards we were taught to "manage symptoms", to suppress them using a vast array of drugs. Or surgery. Or radiation. It was taboo to ask why people got ill, and it was taboo to use the words "healing" or "cure". The names of the main categories of drugs began – begin – with the prefix "anti": anti-inflammatories, anti-biotics, anti-epileptics, anti-psychotics, anti-hypertensives, anti-histamines, anti-emetics, anti-depressants, and so on ad infinitum. There was a sense of fighting the body's processes, not getting alongside the body as an ally. There was no concept of strengthening the immune system so it could fight its own battles. There was no wondering, simply, what the body was missing – what it might need.

As a junior doctor in general medicine, surgery and A&E, my sense was that all the patients we saw were already seriously ill, and that intervention to help them should have happened much, much earlier. It was not until the 1990s that I discovered a society of doctors who were deeply disillusioned with dishing out the "anti" drugs, and who were asking the same questions I had been asking all along. And excitingly, they were finding answers. This was the BSEM, British Society for Ecological Medicine.*

I retrained with their two-year post-grad programme, and was

---

* Back then it was called the BSAENM, British Society for Allergy, Environmental and Nutritional Medicine.

lucky enough to sit in on consultations with many of the most senior practitioners of this new kind of medicine. Eventually, I began to practise Ecological Medicine myself, and now I see patients who have been told for years that nothing can be done getting better. When a doctor tells someone, "There's nothing wrong," they really mean, "I don't know what's wrong. Your symptoms do not fit a pattern in my textbook."

We were not taught in medical school to say, "I don't know." Ever. Now I sometimes have occasion to say to patients: "I don't know what's wrong. Yet. But I am going to find out. We, together, are going to find out." And almost always, we do.

I have lost count of the number of patients who, recovered or recovering, have pleaded with me to write a book about this approach to medicine. My hope is to empower the general public to learn what I and my colleagues, students and patients have learnt about how to get well and stay well.

Ecological Medicine: Principles And Foundations

I learnt a lot of valuable skills and science as a medical student and then as a junior doctor, but everything I will be sharing with you in these pages I have learnt in the past 20 years, practising Ecological Medicine. Ecological Medicine is not a speciality, because it does not restrict itself to one part of the body or one type of disease. It is an approach that sees the whole body as a joined-up ecosystem, and also sees it within the ecosystem of the planet we live on. It looks at how your nutrition and environment are affecting your body and mind, and it focuses on the causes and prevention of illness. It doesn't rely on drugs, and it takes account of the fact that we are all genetically unique, and therefore all biochemically different.

Ecological Medicine begins with believing the patient; if you don't feel right, there **is** a reason. Most of the people whom I help have been told: "all your tests are normal, there is nothing wrong", or some variant of "it's all in your mind". Many of today's most prevalent symptom patterns – illnesses – are not (yet) in the medical textbooks. But they're still real.

In essence, Ecological Medicine has two major aspects: Nutritional Medicine – putting the good stuff back in to the body, and Environmental Medicine – taking the bad stuff out.

Environmental medicine

Let's talk about the "bad stuff" briefly first, as it is not mentioned much in most "how to be healthy" books. In the polluted 21st century, we live surrounded by artificial chemicals which our bodies are not evolved to cope with. Some 80,000–100,000 have been synthesised since the Industrial Revolution. They are in common use, and find their way into our air, water, soil and food, and thence into us. Car fumes, industrial waste, pesticides, heavy metals – we are exposed to all these and many more with very little choice. Then there are the toxic chemicals to which we expose ourselves voluntarily, but in blissful ignorance – our perfume or aftershave, deodorant and hair spray, the kitchen cleaning fluids under the sink, the stain remover, the car oil, the air freshener we spray in the toilet.

All of these substances are alien to the human body, and they accumulate over the years, potentially doing us serious harm.[1,2,3]

One of the many ways they can harm us is by pushing vital nutrients out of the body; hence the need to put the nutrients back in as well as taking the toxins out. This is what detoxification or "detox" should be about; not just a fast or a cleanse for vague and hopeful reasons, but an education about how to minimise our exposure to the unavoidable poisons (detoxification means unpoisoning), and to replace the ones we may choose to use, like perfume, with safe, natural versions.

Nutritional medicine

Now: putting the good stuff in. Regarding nutrition, you will have noticed that there is a bewildering array of food fads and fashions out there, shifting rapidly, and with wildly conflicting messages about what to eat and how to live in order to be healthy. The intention of this book is to steer you safely through and past them all, making nutritional science clear and simple, and enabling you to work out what's needed for you personally to get well and stay well. But first, it is extremely instructive to see **why** there is such a vast and confusing range of nutritional advice around. The vignette that follows will illustrate this:

Sofia is in her kitchen, cooking up the jumbo oats which she soaked last night. She is sprinkling nuts and seeds and berries into the pot. She will have lentils for lunch, brown rice and a seaweed salad for supper. Whatever I think about this, Sofia is happy. Sofia is thrilled. She has been living like this for two months now and her painful arthritic joints have improved spectacularly. She can walk freely; nothing aches.

Ben, on the other side of town, is also having breakfast. He is over the moon with his new (two-months-old) regime; instead of the cereal and toast of his previous life, he is having eggs and bacon, tomatoes and mushroom and sausage. A full English fry-up, just like his grandfather used to have. Ben is overjoyed because his crippling fatigue has gone. He can stay awake all day at work, he can concentrate, he's not reaching for the biscuits at 11.00am or collapsing in a heap at 4.00pm. He's walking home, not sitting on the bus, because he can. His energy has come back.

Sofia and Ben have both been on a nutrition course, but not the same one. They don't know each other. What they have in common is that each of them has found an eating plan that works – for their particular body, for their particular illness and for this particular moment in their life. Sofia and Ben might be so excited about their amazing recoveries that they each publish a book about it, wanting us all to be similarly saved from illness. This is totally understandable, and it is the reason why there is so much confusing advice about what to eat and how to live. It's all mutually contra-dictory, but that doesn't necessarily mean that any of it is actually wrong. Mostly, it is just what has worked for the person who wrote it, at the phase of their life when they wrote it.

But hold on. What if we revisit Sofia and Ben some years later? Oh dear. Sofia's body has run out of Vitamin D reserves, and she has ended up with severe depression.[4] Ben is having investigations for painful stomach problems; he's hoping it isn't cancer. He never did read the ingredients list on his packets of sausages, or check what kind of oil he was cooking his breakfast in.

This book will make it possible for you to find the right eating pattern for yourself, in whatever life phase and situation you find yourself right now. And it will give you the principles of sane, safe and sensible eating, and supplementing if necessary, that you can sustain for life. Any eating plan that strikes you as extreme probably **is** extreme. It may be very useful indeed to some people, for a limited period of time. Fasts and "cleanse plans" do have their place, but only as temporary fixes. (Sofia and Ben didn't realise this.) After such programmes, or indeed instead of them, we have to return to ordinary reality, and find ways of eating and ways of living that are not only healthy but also practical, sustainable and compatible with our everyday lives.

My aim in this book is two-fold: to enable you to feel better now, with an increased level of physical energy and mental clarity, AND to reduce your chances of getting a serious illness in the future. There are a lot of serious illnesses about but, as we'll see, there is loads we can do to prevent them. Here are just a few of our modern epidemics:

Acne
Addictions
ADHD
Allergies
Anxiety
Arthritis
Asthma
Autism and ASD
Auto-immune diseases
Cancer
Chronic Fatigue Syndrome/ME
Dementia
Depression
Diabetes

Eczema
Endometriosis
Fertility problems
Fibroids
Hay Fever
Heart disease
Hyperactivity
Inflammatory Bowel Disease
Irritable Bowel Syndrome
Lupus
Motor Neurone Disease
Multiple Sclerosis
Obesity
Parkinson's Disease
Period problems and PMS
Polycystic ovaries
Stroke
Thyroid problems

And there are many more.

These are 21st century plagues, which were rare or unknown before the industrial revolution. They are **not** inevitable, and they are **not** primarily about ageing. (Cancer, for example, is increasing fastest among children, not adults.) These diseases have causes, to do with our environment, our nutrition and the way we live. That means they are potentially preventable.

But with so many diet plans out there, it's hard not to feel bombarded and bewildered. One of them will tell you to eat no meat, another will tell you to eat loads of meat. One will tell you to live on fruit, another will tell you to avoid fruit like the plague! Among those currently competing for our attention are: Atkins, Cambridge, Dukan, Feingold, Five-two, Fodmaps, Fruitarian, Hay, Ketogenic, Low-histamine, Macrobiotic, Mediterranean, Paleo, Raw food, Sirt, Specific Carbohydrate, South beach, Zone...

Most of them have some really useful elements, but remember: each of them works for somebody, none of them works for everybody, and none of them will work for anybody the whole time! There is no **one** way of eating that's right for all of the people all of the time. How to eat depends on your body (your genes, your metabolism, your hormonal status and your age) and on where you live, how you live, your exercise level and the season. There are, however, some key guiding principles that all of us can use, which I outline later in this chapter. By the end of this book, you'll know what to eat, and how and when, for your *own* health. You'll also have a good sense of how that might change as you grow older, and if you're a parent, you'll learn a lot about how to keep your children healthy.

Seasonality: Why It Matters For Your Health

Should we eat the same foods all the year round? The answer, as you may have guessed, is a resounding No. Our bodies are not the same all the year round. Our nutritional needs change with the changing seasons, and in pre-industrial times we would only have eaten what was available locally and in season. That was not perfect, but it did have some nutritional benefits which we have lost in the era of air-freighting, supermarket shopping and always-being-in-a-hurry.

Firstly, we now expect to have all foods available all year round, and the supermarkets ensure that we keep on expecting this. It is highly profitable for them, but bad for our bodies and bad for the planet. Secondly, we live mostly indoors, with central heating, so that even in winter our bodies may think it is summer. Lastly, climate change means that the seasons have become less clearly defined; often you don't know what season you're in till you wake up in the morning. You can no longer predict the weather just by knowing which month it is on the calendar. I believe this is one of the factors making our bodies disorientated, like bees in electro-smog.

For all these reasons, we have become cut off from the clues in nature that would have told us what we needed to eat. Even to be asking the question, "What should we eat?" would have been unthinkable not so long ago. We ate what grew, when it grew.

The most glaring example is fruit. In the UK, berries ripen in the summer, and apples and pears ripen in the autumn. That's when it's good to eat them. If you are eating all types of fruit, every day, all the year round, then three harmful things are happening:

1 You are simply eating fruit of poorer quality. Fruit that's local and in season tastes better because it **is** better; it is fresh, so it contains all the nutrients and flavours it is meant to contain, especially Vitamin C; it doesn't just taste of water and sugar.

2 You are putting a continuous dose of sugar into your gut, thus promoting the growth of yeasts and unfriendly bacteria (more on this in Chapter 2).

3 Aeroplanes are flying that fruit across the globe from the southern hemisphere, contributing to climate change and causing much of the pollution which, as I describe in Chapter 7, is making so many of us ill.

The first four chapters of this book are each about one particular season, and how to stay healthy in that season. Each of these season-based chapters will tell you:

🌿 What food is in season and good to eat

🌿 What's out of season and not worth eating

🌿 Which nutrients you might be lacking at this time of year, and what to do about that

🌿 Specific health hazards of that season, and how to prevent them

🌿 Case histories to illustrate the above (all the case histories in this book have been disguised sufficiently to protect the identity of the patient)

🌿 Take-home tips for staying well in that particular season

I am writing from a UK perspective, although the principles apply wherever in the world you live. However, there is one seasonal issue that applies specifically to temperate zones: the changing rhythms of the *day* with the different times of the year. This is about light and dark, and it has real implications for our health and well-being. And, unlike the temperature, it won't change with global warming, so long as the Earth keeps turning.

Got to get up at 5.00am for work? That's perfectly fine and natural in June. But having to do it in December can make you ill. Hiding under the duvet at 5.00pm? That makes perfect sense in January. It's dark. Stay there, guilt-free! But if you're doing it in mid-summer, something may be wrong.

The pineal gland in our brain responds to light and dark, and we ignore it at our peril. I know most of us have little choice about the way we live (which is why the term "lifestyle" is so unfair and irritating). But to the extent that it's possible for you, adjust the rhythm of your day according to the light/dark cycle. We are "designed" to hibernate in winter to a great extent, and to play and party outdoors in summer. Schools and work places ignore this geo-biological rhythm completely, and we all suffer as a result. Changing the clocks twice a year is irrelevant; we need to try and *live* differently at the different times of the year.

The evolutionary perspective

In trying to figure out what on earth to eat, and in navigating our way through the maze of contradictory advice, an evolutionary perspective can be very useful. It asks us to consider how our bodies have developed over the long, slow process of evolution, and reminds us that compared to our millions of years living in forests and caves, the past 10,000 years of agriculture are but a fleeting moment, and the most recent 250 years of industrialisation are briefer still.

The body and its physiological needs and responses have barely changed at all since we were hunter-gatherers living in nomadic tribes, foraging for food in the wild. Biological adaptation to a changing environment (by Darwinian natural selection) is an incredibly slow process, but our environment – and our food – have altered at break neck pace in recent centuries. Our bodies simply haven't been able to keep up.

So here we are, feeling ill or worn out, or simply not as well as we know we could be, and the evolutionary perspective comes along and says: "Well, let's eat the food our bodies were 'designed' to eat – the kind of food our hunter-gatherer ancestors ate."[5] It sounds sensible, and I believe it can be a very useful guide. Only a guide, though, not a religion! In working out what's the healthiest way for YOU to eat, therefore, the evolutionary perspective should have a vote, but not a veto. The veto, the final decision about how to eat, lies with your body. No one else's body, no one else's theory. (For more on this see "Suck It And See" on page 33.)

Shortly, I'll outline some ways in which the evolutionary perspective can be really helpful. But first, how do we really know what our hunter-gatherer ancestors ate? This is what I call the "Paleo Problem", as in Paleolithic, Old Stone Age. People talk about the Stone Age diet, but what do they think they mean?

Well, there are two main sorts of evidence. Firstly, archaeology: bits of ancient food preserved, remarkably, inside the remains of our distant ancestors. What the fossil record shows us is that our hunter-gatherer forbears had one major feature in their diet that we lack – namely, huge variety. Wherever they lived, they ate literally thousands of different foods, both plant and animal. There was, of course, much greater biodiversity, and they ate whatever they could pick or catch. In season, naturally. With the advent of farming, the range became narrower, and with industrialised agribusiness, narrower still.

How many different species of vegetable do you eat in a year? Your ancient ancestors could add two zeroes to that figure. One of the reasons that food allergies have become so common is simply that people are eating the same foods, day in, day out. In China they are developing allergies to rice, in the UK to wheat, in the USA to maize/sweetcorn. "Staple" foods are bad news; your body gets literally sick of eating the same stuff all the time. It's monocrop farming, so it's monocrop eating. Bad for the soil, bad for us. Great for unfriendly bugs and pests, both in the fields and in our intestines.

The second source of evidence for what our ancestors ate comes from the study of surviving hunter-gatherer tribes. This is where the picture becomes rather more complicated. Some people believe that these tribal peoples chase wild animals all day, and then eat them, and live on plants, nuts and very occasional fruits in between the meat-feasts. In other words, that they eat virtually no carbohydrates, and certainly no grains. But let's look more closely, as this is not always the case.

The Yanomami people, for example, are a tribe who live deep in the South American rainforest.[6] They do hunt game and gather plants, but they also grind cassava roots into flour and make bread from them. Similarly, the Tsimané people who live in the Amazon in Bolivia eat a mixture of sweetcorn, cassava (again), rice and plantain – that's all carbohydrate – plus the *small* amount of game and fish that they catch. The Tsimané are among the healthiest people on the planet[7] – no heart disease, strokes or diabetes etc. – although sadly this is already starting to change as the relentless progress of Western "civilisation" has begun to encroach on their land and their lives.

There is a current fashion to eat no carbs, partly because it is thought that this is how tribal peoples live. In fact, tribal peoples eat plenty of carbs, but – here's the catch – they also walk or run for six to eight hours most days, chasing their preferred dinner. If we did that, we could probably get away with eating loads of carbs too.

And here's a caveat; present-day tribal peoples who have survived into the 21st century may not in fact be wholly representative of what most ancient humans ate. This is because they now occupy only the most inhospitable places on the planet,[8] the tiny enclaves which have not been colonised. Our ancestors may have had it easier than the Yanomami and Tsimané.

What did your ancient ancestors eat? A seasonally available mixture of meat, fish (if they were near the sea or a lake or river), plants, nuts, seeds and seedlings, roots, tubers and occasional fruit. One thing we can be sure of, though, is that it was not the same as the food that **my** ancient ancestors ate, because they lived in different places.

Even today, if you compare the average diet in southern India, say, with the typical diet in Greenland, you'll find it to be very, very different. Just as you need different food in different seasons, you need different food in different countries. In fact, if you want to know how to eat in a cold winter, study the Inuit peoples. If you want to know how to eat in a hot summer, check out the Indian way. Remember Sofia on page 5? She would have been alright, eating her vegan diet, for rather longer in India than she was in the UK. She would have got all the Vitamin D she needed from the sunshine.

In hot countries, people tend to save the main meal of the day till evening; it's simply too hot to be hungry earlier in the day. So, should we do that in a British summer? No. Because in hot countries people (still, mostly) have a siesta; they sleep in the afternoon. That means they can stay up late, hours after their evening meal, without sleep deprivation. They get time to digest. They are not going to bed on a full stomach – a thing one should never do – but in Britain a large meal at 9.00pm is way, way too late. In cold countries people tend to eat their main meal much earlier in the day. Again, it makes sense; they need food to fuel them through the day in a cold climate.

The most useful aspect of the evolutionary perspective is that it can help us resolve the important how-to-eat dilemmas that are all over the press and plaguing so many of us. Questions like, for my health, should I be:

Vegan? Vegetarian? Pescatarian? Carnivorous? Fruitarian? Eat raw food only?

The answer is, it depends on where you live, the climate, the season, and all the factors that make your own body unique, as mentioned above. So, who was closer to a true Stone Age diet, Sofia or Ben? Both and neither. Stone-age people would have sometimes eaten like Sofia (but without the porridge, rice or lentils) and, when they could, more like Ben (without the artificial additives). But they would never have eaten one way only, repetitively, all year round. So here's a suggestion for how to eat in the 21st century:

- December, January, February: Be a carnivore.

- March, April, May: Be a vegetarian.

- June, July, August: Be a vegan.

- September, October, November: Be a pescatarian (eat fish but not meat).

That's an idea, not a rigid prescription, but it offers a way to eat, and to think about eating, that provides a good balance for the planet as well as for the individual; usually, what's good for the planet is good for the person. Now let's look at the implications of some of these different ways of eating.

A word about meat-eating:
The higher up the evolutionary ladder an animal is – the closer it is to us – the more "a little goes a long way", for our bodies and for the planet. In other words, if we're going to eat mammals (red meat) we should do so infrequently, maybe once a week or once a fortnight rather than several times a week. The studies showing that increased red meat consumption increased cancer rates, by the way, were not done with people eating organically reared meat.[9,10] So they were effectively looking at the results of eating pesticides, antibiotics and hormones, rather than meat per se. They also didn't allow for how many vegetables their subjects were (or weren't) consuming.

But hey – those of us who do eat meat are **wasting** most of the animal! We cut off the fat, thereby losing the vital, fat-soluble vitamins A, D, E and K. We throw out the highly nutritious liver, heart, kidneys and brain, calling it "offal". We chuck out the adrenal gland, which contains Vitamin C; that's how the traditional Inuit and other northern peoples got their Vitamin C in the long Arctic winter, by eating the whole seal, adrenal gland and all. If we went back to using the whole animal, we could also eat fewer animals. And please note: carnivores still need to eat vegetables – lots of them. We cannot live by meat alone.

A word about fish-eating:

We evolved from the sea, and we need what grows in the sea. Fish contain vitamins A, D and B2 (Riboflavin), many minerals including the vital mineral iodine, omega 3 essential fatty acids (good for your brain) and easily digested protein. Fish also, sadly, contain some of the pollution we have put into the sea, which builds up through the food chain, so that bigger fish (like tuna) contain more toxins than little fish (like sardines). On balance, I believe it's still safer to eat some fish than no fish, especially as by the end of this book you will know how to get the toxins out of your system. But we urgently need to clean up our oceans.

A word about being vegetarian:

This means that you do eat eggs and dairy produce, but no meat or fish. It's ok for most people, so long as they eat plenty of eggs (yes I said plenty of eggs; if you are worried about cholesterol, check out Dr Malcolm Kendrick's book *The Great Cholesterol Con* or the work of Justin Smith). But not too much dairy produce;

good-quality cheese and butter and yogurt are alright for most people, but milk isn't. Milk is food that nature designed for baby mammals of the same species, not for adult mammals of a different species. Cow's milk is great for calves, but not for us. Many of my vegetarian patients have developed dairy allergies, by overdoing the dairy products. Why are they craving dairy? Because their body is telling them they need some animal protein. Just a little, from time to time. If they feel able to follow that prompting, and eat just a little fish or free-range, organic meat now and then, their felt need for excess dairy products goes away.

There is a particular type of vegetarianism that permits dairy products but not eggs. This is usually for cultural/religious reasons, so when patients come to me eating like this, I cannot change it. But what does help is to choose your dairy products with care. For thousands of years, humans have been turning animal milk into something far more digestible for adult humans: cheese, butter, yogurt, curds and whey. If it is raw – unpasteurised – so much the better; less likely to cause all the excess mucus and sinus trouble and general snottiness that too much dairy products can lead to. Please ensure it's organic, so you are not eating pesticides, antibiotics and synthetic hormones, about which more shortly.

For some people, goat's or sheep's "dairy" products are far less allergenic than cow's dairy. To find out if this is true for you, just Suck it and See – cut out **all** dairy products for 2 weeks, then try goat's butter/cheese/yogurt (one per day, not all at once) and see what happens. Then sheep's. Then buffalo and camel if you want! But don't waste your pennies on expensive blood tests for food allergy; it's more scientific to find out for yourself. For more details on how to do it, see "An Elimination Diet" for detecting food allergy, pages 135–140, in Becky's case history.

A word about being vegan:

Vegans eat no animal products at all; no meat, fish, eggs or dairy. The strictest vegans eat no honey (it exploits the bees) and won't wear leather shoes. It is fine for a while. It is fine for longer in a hot country where you get all your Vitamin D simply from the action of sunlight on bare skin. It is fine as a temporary "cleanse". But not everyone can live on plants alone indefinitely. Unlike cows and sheep, we humans do not have a ruminant's gut; we have only one stomach.

Long-term vegans miss out on iron and Vitamin B12; that much is well-known. They also, as I've said, miss out on Vitamin D if they live in a cold and cloudy place like the UK. They may also – this is less well-known – miss out on the amino acids carnitine,[11] taurine[12] and tryptophan[13] and others. Carnitine is vital for transporting fatty acids into mitochondria (organelles within the cell) for energy production, and taurine is vital for the function of the brain and the heart, and for making bile for our digestive systems. Tryptophan gets converted into serotonin, the "happiness hormone", or more accurately the happiness neurotransmitter. Vegans may also miss out on Vitamin A, which is found only in animal foods. Most vegans will convert beta-carotene from vegetables into Vitamin A, as we all do,[14] but not everyone converts at the same rate, and some long-term vegans may not make enough Vitamin A to keep their eyes healthy.

Crucially, and perhaps surprisingly, vegans miss out on some essential minerals which **are** contained in plant food, but are not well **absorbed** from plant food. So my vegan patients are often astonished to discover, on nutritional blood-testing, that they are desperately low in the vital minerals zinc and magnesium. "But I eat loads of pumpkin seeds and sunflower seeds!" they exclaim. "Those are full of zinc and magnesium!"

Indeed they are. But – how can I put this delicately? – the sunflower seeds and pumpkin seeds may just come out the other end. Not every human digestive tract can break them down and digest them and extract the minerals from them in sufficient quantity to meet our nutritional needs. Some can. These are the healthy vegans; I don't see them as patients. What I do see is that among my patients with ME/Chronic Fatigue Syndrome, 80–90% are either vegan, or they are second generation vegetarian, by which I mean a life-long vegetarian born to a mother who was also vegetarian all her adult life.

I work with them to improve their gut function (see Chapter 2), maximising the potential of their small intestine to extract the vital nutrients out of their plant food. It helps. But those who make the most clinical improvement are those who decide to introduce into their diet, now and then, a little bit of sustainably caught fish, or a little bit of free-range, humanely reared, organic poultry. As soup if necessary, if they feel they just cannot chew flesh.

It has to be said, the vegans' fierce critique of cruel factory-farming methods is correct; but we don't need to eat that kind of meat. There are alternatives now, on which more below.

Even though your soul may be vegan, your body may be a carnivore. At least occasionally. We evolved as omnivores, eating a little bit of everything, but not an overdose of anything.

Guidelines for 99 per cent of us

Of course we're all unique, and our food needs will vary according to our genetics, metabolism, hormonal status, age, gender, activity level, where we live and the season. BUT there are a few basic rules, in addition to "Eat what's naturally in season" that do apply to all of us. Here are my **4 golden rules**:

1 Eat your greens
2 Cut out sugar
3 Cut out artificial additives
4 Eat organic and free-range, i.e. real food

Now, to elaborate on each of these, and the reasons for them:

1 **Eat your greens!** Simple as that. Grandma was right. Green leafy vegetables such as spinach, cabbage, broccoli, pak choi, watercress, lettuce and so on have at least three huge benefits. First, they make a clean sweep through the digestive tract, carrying all before them. They act like a gentle broom, ensuring that your intestines move properly and nothing gets stuck. Sorry to be graphic, but the fact is, if you can poo properly, regularly and comfortably, you can be healthy and think clearly. This has been known forever, but needs repeating.[15]

Second huge benefit: green leaves contain many essential nutrients, including the vital mineral magnesium, one atom of which sits at the heart of each molecule of chlorophyll (the substance that makes plants green).

Thirdly, green veg in general and the brassica family in

particular (broccoli, cabbage, kale, Brussels sprouts and cauliflower) have been shown to be protective against cancer.[16]

Should you have your green leafy veg raw or cooked? Both! Raw means that the Vitamin C and other antioxidants are not destroyed. Cooked means that your gut will be better able to absorb the magnesium and other minerals. Digestion-wise, it's best to have salad at lunch and cooked veg at dinner. And, of course, seasonally, to have more salad in summer and more cooked veg in winter. Beyond that, people vary widely with regard to what's the best ratio of raw-to-cooked food for them.

The raw-food fanatics advocate a diet of only raw foods. Guess what – it worked for **them**! The macrobiotics people insist that **all** our food should be cooked. Guess what – (etc.). The Ayurvedic approach (Indian herbal medicine; long and venerable tradition) says that different people need different ratios of raw-to-cooked food. Hallelujah. They have an elaborate diagnostic system for finding out which type you are. It's pretty reliable actually. But you could just suck it and see – and be guided by the seasons and times of day, as above.

There is a recipe for green vegetable juice in Chapter 7 and for salad dressing (for raw greens) in Chapter 3. For cooking your greens, please, please don't ever boil them. Sauté them in organic coconut oil, with garlic and onion and herbs. Or maybe steam them lightly. But don't boil them; it kills them, it kills your appetite for them, it stinks the kitchen out, it puts the kids off for life, and the Vitamin C

and the taste go down the drain with the water. Promise?
Thank you.

2 **Cut out the sugar!** Not all carbs. Just sugar. This is not news.
Professor John Yudkin wrote *Pure, White and Deadly* back in
1962. Since that time, sugar hasn't become any less deadly,
even though much of it is now brown. Whatever its colour, it
still rots your teeth and gums, feeds the least friendly bugs in
your gut (see Chapter 2), and contributes mightily to diabetes,
obesity and many more diseases. Sugar uses up your minerals
and vitamins too; it is an "anti-nutrient".

Sugar is a major causative factor in heart disease as well,
but for over 40 years the margarine manufacturers found it
profitable to claim that the big baddie was animal fat. It isn't
– unless you're a rabbit.

John Yudkin's truth-telling back then was very
inconvenient for the sugar industry, and made him very
unpopular. When I was a junior doctor back in the early
1980s, the "Sugar Board" regularly sent us promotional
material, explaining that sugar was totally safe because it was
"**natural**". It is well worth examining this claim, because it is
still being used to mislead and confuse us today. Sugar is a
natural substance, yes. That is, it occurs naturally in plants,
particularly in roots, tubers, grains and fruits. Plants
manufacture it. So what's the problem?

The problem is quantity. Concentration. Again, the
evolutionary perspective helps us to understand this. In our
original, natural state, as hunter-gatherers, we would have had
access only very rarely to sweet foods. Fruit and berries

would have been occasional treats, usually in autumn, when they helped us lay down fat for the coming winter, in temperate climates. Perhaps a cave-man or cave-woman would have found honey once in a lifetime, getting badly stung in the process and never trying again (as in Winnie the Pooh).

BUT nature has primed us to crave and consume sweet, sugary foods – it's a survival mechanism adapted for an environment where food of all sorts was scarce. It was very helpful back then to have the occasional fruit-feast, when our most nutritious food was something we had to run 20 miles to catch. Furthermore, breast-milk is sweet, so the sweet taste is associated with safety and love and comfort at a primal level, for all of us.

But today this in-built sugar craving has become a liability, in an environment full of tempting, easily available, instant, cheap and highly concentrated sugar. It's there by the supermarket check-out, and disguised as a protein bar in the health-food shop. It's in many processed and packaged foods, even savoury ones; any ingredient ending with the suffix "-ose" is a sugar. They sneak it in to make the food addictive. Sugar is ubiquitous.

As Professor Robert Lustig points out in his brilliant book *Fat Chance*, willpower alone will not cure you of craving sugar; it's programmed in. But there are many things we **can** do to stop ourselves overdosing on the sweet stuff.

The first one is: Stop Feeling Guilty! It's not your fault. You're not weak-willed. The problem is not you, it is our sugar-loaded environment. The second thing to do is to start switching your taste buds over "from sweet to green" –

introduce the opposite flavours into your diet, and let your taste buds get used to them. So try grapefruits and blackcurrants – sour. Dark green leafy veg like kale and spinach – bitter. At least, they may taste bitter at first if you're not used to them. Learn to love them. This can help to make sugar taste TOO sweet, and even sickly; you'll start to notice what an over-the-top flavour it actually is.

Then treat withdrawing from sugar as you would withdrawing from any addictive drug; do it according to temperament. If you are an all-or-nothing person, you may choose to go "cold turkey" and just stop. If you are more of a "gently does it" type, you will want to withdraw more gradually. But either way, you will need to identify where sugar is hiding in processed foods, as above.

Don't starve yourself; the commonest reason for a sugar binge is simply getting too hungry, forgetting to eat, being too busy to eat. Once hunger goes past a certain point, you will just go straight for the sugar. You can prevent this by remembering to eat regular meals. Lastly, remember it is not just you who is craving sugar, it is the Trillions of Tiny Companions in your gut – lots more on this in Chapter 2. Once you have sorted them out ("How to Spring Clean Your Gut", pages 82–92) the craving will be much less intense, and you will even be able to indulge in the sweet stuff occasionally without getting "hooked" again.

3 **Cut out all artificial additives – they are not food!** If you were dyeing a tee-shirt, you wouldn't suck the dye, would you? But our kids are eating blue ice-lollies; they're eating

toxic dyes. People who work in the printing-and-dyeing industry are prone to bladder cancer;[17] this is well recognised. But manufacturers are allowed to put artificial colours in our food, despite the known dangers.[18,19]

Then there are artificial flavours. Why should a food product need artificial flavouring, if not to disguise the fact that it's rubbish? And there's a loophole in the food-labelling laws that allows food producers to just write "flavouring", without telling you what the chemical actually is. It may well be carcinogenic – but you can't look it up and find out.

Then there's "natural flavouring". This is usually a con, and an abuse of the much-abused word "natural". Arsenic is natural. Petrol is natural – it is made from crude oil which comes from the decay of million-year-old dead trees. But you wouldn't drink it, and you get sick from inhaling or handling it too much. Ultimately, everything is natural, because even the most synthetic substance created in a factory is made from raw materials found on Planet Earth, because that's all we have. But factory processes can turn ingredients that were indeed harmless in their original form into something toxic, by the way the molecules are altered, combined, heated and damaged; this is particularly important with respect to fats and oils (see pp 323–325).

"Emulsifiers" are another common type of food additive. They allow oils and water to mix (which they don't do on their own) to create a smooth, creamy texture that the food industry has decreed we should like, and then claims we "demand".

Artificial sweeteners abound. Aspartame, Acesulfame K,

Sucralose and so on are the latest dangerous incarnation; Cyclamates and Saccharin were banned years ago, but have quietly crept back onto the menu, despite their toxic potential.[20,21,22,23,24,25]

When we eat sugar, our pancreas gland produces insulin, to transport the sugar out of our bloodstream and into our cells. We used to think that our blood level of insulin rose just in response to a rise in blood sugar level. But now it seems that insulin secretion also responds directly to a sweet taste on the tongue[26] – and these sweeteners are many times sweeter than sugar. So even completely artificial, calorie-free sweeteners may trigger this rise, as the body is anticipating a rush of actual sugar into the blood, and the job of insulin is to lower blood sugar levels.

When insulin goes ahead and does its job, in the absence of any actual sugar, you may feel faint and hungry (hypoglycaemia). So you may overeat an hour or two after swallowing the artificial sweetener. This could well be one of the reasons why artificial sweeteners don't help people to lose weight, and they don't reverse or prevent diabetes.[27]

"Natural" sweeteners such as Xylitol and Stevia will, I predict, turn out to be problematic too. Similarly with agave syrup, date syrup, rice syrup etc. They Are Just Sugar, extracted from agave, dates and rice respectively. As above, what is unnatural about them is their concentration; more actual sugar in one hit than our forest-dwelling ancestors got in a whole year. There is no substitute for retraining your taste buds!

Trans fats and hydrogenated fats should count as artificial

additives too; their risks to health are well-known (see references 246–251), and some manufacturers are removing them, but not all; read the label carefully.

There are hundreds of food additives out there, but you get the gist: avoid them. There are a couple of exceptions, though. "Tocopherol" is Vitamin E, and "Ascorbic Acid" is Vitamin C. They are used as antioxidants to stop food going off, in the same way they prevent toxic oxidation in our own bodies. So they're ok. But most additives are junk, not food. Best not to feed them to your children, or yourself.

Keeping a food diary

In regard to eventually eliminating both sugar and artificial additives, you may find it useful to keep a food diary for a week or so. Just five columns: breakfast, lunch, dinner, snacks and drinks. Write down whatever you eat and drink. Don't beat yourself up about it; this is not a judgement exercise. It's just for your own information; we can be so busy we don't actually realise what we're eating, or not eating, till we look back over a week's record. Did you miss meals? Is your snacks column full of sugar? We can't begin to change things till we've noticed them.

4 **Eat free-range, organic food.** "Free-range" applies to animal food, "organic" applies to both plant and animal food. Let's talk about free-range first — what it is and why it matters.

Free-range animals are free to roam around on the grass. They are not penned in. The cows can graze, the hens can peck. In the case of hens, they have a shelter to go into at night, to be safe from foxes, but it's not a cramped torture-chamber like the places where battery hens are kept. If it's not free-range, it's a battery chicken; it's factory-farmed. Don't buy it. This matters equally whether you're eating the egg or eating the chicken. And with regard to cows, it matters equally whether you're eating dairy products or beef.

So, in so far as it's possible, those of us who eat meat need to try to be compassionate carnivores. But eating free-range is not only about being more ethical. It's also better for your health. A free, happy animal is going to be digesting and excreting properly. It's less likely to have an infection, because happy animals have stronger immune systems. And it's not full of the stress hormones cortisol and adrenaline.

Now, organic. Yes, I know it's more expensive; I'll address that in a minute. First, I want to explain what it is and why it really, really matters.

Organic food isn't some kind of weird, different, special food. It's ORDINARY food, food like our great-grandparents ate. Without pesticides, synthetic hormones or antibiotics in it. What **is** weird is food that's full of pesticides, synthetic hormones and antibiotics! That's artificial food. And it's everywhere.

Organic food is simply food that **hasn't** been sprayed with pesticides, **hasn't** been injected with synthetic hormones and **hasn't** been fed on antibiotics. That's all. It should, of course, be the norm – as it used to be. But sadly, most plant crops these days are treated with weed-killers and insecticides. Cows and pigs are often injected with synthetic hormones, used as growth promoters; this is not allowed by the EU, but in the UK at least 30% of our meat is imported from countries where it **is** allowed – and that percentage is about to rise. Furthermore, hens, cows and pigs are often fed on continual antibiotics, creating risky, antibiotic-resistant infections in the animals themselves, and in us if we eat them.

This is big, profitable, mass-scale agribusiness: bad for the land, for the animals and for us. Spraying the crops makes life more convenient for farm owners; that's why they do it. But pesticides are chemicals closely related to nerve gas; they can damage our nervous system, endocrine system, reproductive system, immune system and more. They have made some farmers very ill too[28,29,30] – those who do the actual spraying. Similarly with sheep dipping.

Putting hormones into cows makes them grow fatter and faster. But these hormones are implicated in the rise of breast cancer, prostate cancer and obesity in humans. If we eat the meat or dairy produce of such animals, we are eating those hormones as well, and they work as growth-promoters in us too, encouraging the excess proliferation of cells in our hormone-sensitive tissues, e.g. breast and prostate. And their effect will be combined with that of the pesticides, which are both carcinogens and EDCs (Endocrine Disrupting Compounds).

Why are antibiotics routinely fed to farm animals? Well, they say it's to prevent infection. But it's interesting that free-range, organically reared animals very rarely get infections; it is only factory-farmed creatures, their immune systems weakened by distress (and by the poor-quality food they're given) which succumb en masse to infection. Remember BSE (Mad Cow Disease)? Cows that were reared completely organically from birth didn't get it; they were never fed on the macerated remains of their fellow-creatures.[31]

In the old days, farmers called the vet if a beast got sick. Now they keep thousands of birds or mammals crowded together in inhumane conditions which make them sick, and use antibiotics daily as prophylaxis. Not safe, not sustainable.

Eating free-range, organic food means that you don't participate in this inhumanity, and you're not consuming pesticides, synthetic hormones or antibiotics. These chemicals get concentrated up the food chain, so an animal fed on non-organic crops contains even more of whatever-was-sprayed-on-the-crop than the plant crop itself does. Look for the "Soil Association" logo; it means that fruit/veg/grains/beans/nuts are truly organic, and that the cheese/yogurt/butter/eggs/poultry/meat are both organic (i.e. from animals fed only on organic food) and genuinely free-range.

But it's so expensive! Three responses to that. First, what proportion of our income do we spend on food? The Office for National Statistics says that in 1957 we spent 33% of our income on food. By 2006 it was down to 15%, and Professor Chris Elliot, who investigated the "Horsegate" burger scandal, says that it's now only 10%. A fraction. Somehow, we have to readjust, to shift our priorities. Becoming too ill to work drains the finances more than eating organic does.

Second response: with regard to organic, free-range meat and poultry, the way to be able to afford it is simply to eat less of it. Instead of chemical-saturated battery chicken or beef or pork five times a week, try the free-range organic version but only once or twice a week. Better for the planet as well as for your pocket.

Third response: it **shouldn't** be more expensive to eat safe food, it should be cheaper. So write to your MP, and demand to know why the government is subsidising the big chemical farmers when they should be supporting the hard-working, conscientious, good-for-the-soil and good-for-our-health organic farmers.

Suck It And See!

"One person's meat is another person's poison", "Horses for courses", "It takes all sorts", "Each to their own"... the simplest way to find out which eating pattern is best for YOU – at this point in your life, at this time of year – is to experiment. But there are a couple of things you need to know beforehand:

Experimenting with different ways of eating will only work for you, i.e. will only give you the information you need about what's truly most nourishing for your body and brain right now, if you have been following the basic guidelines above. That is, the four golden rules, plus seasonality. For at least four weeks. So check out the chapter for the season you're in right now, and if sugar craving is an issue for you, look up how to deal with it (pages 24–26). Only then will your experiment be valid.

This is because craving and need are very different things. If you have been eating sugar, additives, pesticides etc., and not having enough real food in general and fresh veg in particular, your body will lie to you. People don't **need** doughnuts or MSG-filled takeaways, but as long as they eat them, they will want them; they are made to be addictive. So once you have cut out the junk, your body will start to give you far more accurate messages about what it actually needs. Your intuition will start to lead you towards the foods you need right now, foods that contain the specific nutrients you are lacking. Equally, you will begin to get clearer messages about what is **not** right for you; certain foods may disagree with you and contribute to symptoms of ill health, but you can't figure that out when you're eating rubbish and feeling rubbish every day.

Something like this process occurs naturally in small children and pregnant women – the body gives loud, clear messages about what is right for it and what is wrong for it at that moment. One patient of mine, a young woman with a small baby, was desperately deficient in zinc. When I gave her some zinc drops to take, she reported that her baby – six months old and covered in eczema – had started grabbing the bottle and drinking the zinc! He knew what he needed. (His eczema cleared up, by the way.)

But even in small children and pregnant women, this process of intuition gets distorted by eating sugar, MSG and other addictive substances that are not real food. Eating pure, healthy foods allows the body to tell you what it needs, specifically and clearly. Junk food clouds and covers up those messages.

There is a more formal, controlled version of "Suck it and See", for people who suspect that actual food allergy may be part of their problem, and this method is described under "An Elimination Diet" on pages 135. But even if you are not doing a full-blown elimination diet, do remember to **record** your responses to different foods as you try them out; if you don't jot it down, it's remarkably easy to forget.

Lastly, if changing your eating pattern hasn't helped you feel better, remember that we do breathe as well as eat; are you inhaling something toxic at work? At home? In the street? More on this in Chapter 7.

Case History: Emma's Exhaustion

Emma was 39 when she came to see me, suffering from fatigue, headaches, muscle aches, "brain fog" and frequent coughs and colds. She had three pre-teen children, all boys, and the middle one had special needs. Emma spent a lot of her time and energy battling with her local authority to get this son's educational needs half-met. She also looked after her mother, who was only 70 but had Alzheimer's disease. Emma's husband worked away a lot, so she was effectively single-parenting for most of the week. Lastly, she worked three days a week as a teaching assistant. Unsurprisingly, she was "run down", and catching every virus going round.

Emma's GP had diagnosed her with TATT, which stands for "tired all the time". Emma knew that already. He had quite rightly checked her haemoglobin, thyroid and blood glucose levels; all normal. He told her there was nothing wrong with her, and that she should "just relax". Her reply cannot be printed.

Emma was "Mrs Exhausted Everywoman". Could Nutritional Medicine really help her, when it was clearly her *life* (not life-*style*, because not much choice there) that was draining her? Yes – but it would not be quick or simple.

The low levels of nutrients I found were inextricably linked to Emma's relentlessly demanding life, and we knew that to make her better we were going to have to break that vicious circle. Here's how we did it:

First, the B vitamins. All of them are needed for energy production in the body, and for clear thinking. And we use them up far more rapidly when we are stressed, overtired, doing too much. So Emma's need was greater than average. I prescribed her a B-complex that contained all the B vitamins in serious amounts (mostly 50 mg of each B vitamin), with no additives, and suggested she take one at breakfast and one at lunch. But none in the evening, because most of the B vitamins are "wake you up" nutrients, not conducive to sleep.

Then, Vitamin D. Emma didn't get much sunshine; money was tight, and travelling abroad with the middle child was just too stressful. And although she ate some fish and dairy, it clearly wasn't enough to give her a normal Vitamin D level. So I prescribed that as well, ensuring that it was Vitamin D3, the natural form that the sun makes out of the cholesterol under our skin, and not D2, which is largely synthetic and useless.

Zinc and selenium are both needed for the immune system, specifically for the white blood cells that help us fight infections. Emma was catching every passing bug because her zinc and selenium were low, but equally, every time she caught a cough or cold, the zinc and selenium in her system were being used up by her white blood cells, busy fighting those infections. So that was another vicious circle, and we broke it by giving her good-quality zinc and selenium supplements, again, without needless additives.

The last nutrient that tested low was magnesium. I measure it in the red blood cells, not the plasma, because that is a more accurate reflection of the body's stores. It was spectacularly low. Again, when we are stressed and crazily busy like Emma, we **lose** magnesium. We pee it out. This is an unhelpful biological glitch that may have served a purpose once, but works against us in today's rush-around world. Then, when our magnesium level becomes low, our muscles tense up. Muscles need calcium in order to contract, and magnesium in order to relax. It is physically impossible to relax your muscles (and therefore your self) when your magnesium level is as low as Emma's was. So you get into yet another vicious circle: tense muscles → stress → magnesium loss.

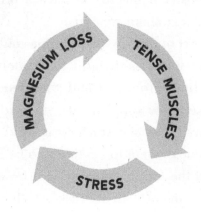

I discussed with Emma how best to raise her magnesium levels. I didn't want to load her with yet more supplements, and in any case, the best way to get substantial amounts of magnesium back into the body is via the skin, by putting Epsom salts in the bath. (Much more on Epsom salts baths in Chapter 7.) But Emma said there was no way she'd have time or "head-space" for that; by the time she'd got all the boys to bed she was "ready to collapse", and didn't want to risk falling asleep in the bath. She said she'd happily swallow a couple more capsules, so I gave her some magnesium to take at bedtime, as that's the best time to take a muscle-relaxant nutrient. (She needed to eat more leafy green veg, full of magnesium, but we were still at the first-aid stage.)

Of course, ideally Emma needed to change her diet; but she was in the Sandwich Generation in two senses, caring for both her mother and her children, and living on sandwiches that she grabbed while rushing from A to B to C. She didn't need me to tell her that this was less than perfect, and she told me clearly that while she cooked for the boys, and usually had their leftovers for supper, she wasn't managing to have a proper breakfast or lunch, and that wasn't about to shift.

Healing is the "Art of the Possible". Emma couldn't abandon her life and disappear to a health farm for a month, much as she would have benefitted from rest and good food and a massage. But she could take a few supplements, she said. She put a chart on her kitchen wall and she stuck to it. And in any case, her nutritional deficiencies were too extreme to be remedied by food alone; she needed the supplements, at least for a while. Although she did also need some protein at breakfast; that really was essential for her energy levels.

When I saw Emma four months later, her muscle aches had gone – that's the magnesium. She hadn't had a cough or cold – that's the Vitamin C, Vitamin D, zinc and selenium. She still often had headaches at the end of the day, but no longer every day. And although she was still physically very tired, she said her "brain fog" was clearing. She could think straight.

Another four months on, the headaches were "rare, and only when I've been super-stressed out about my mum or my middle son". Emma's ability to think clearly was sustained, as were the other improvements, but she was still tired. However, she had decided that she could, after all, find some time on a Saturday to spend cooking. She made healthy meals and froze them, so she had real food at least once a day, through the week. She realised that she could in fact grab a salad along with her sandwich at lunchtime. And she was waking up with a clearer head and a little bit more energy, so she could make a proper breakfast.

The vicious cycles were gradually being replaced by virtuous circles. Once Emma became able to improve her diet, her energy finally improved. Woman cannot live by supplements alone. She is now fit and well and active, and describes her energy level as normal. And she's learnt some useful tips to help her mum and her middle son too.

Health Isn't Just About Nutrition, And Nutrition Isn't Just About Food!

Your health isn't only about your nutrition. It is also, as you probably know already, about fresh air (*clean* fresh air – there's a challenge!), exercise, sleep, avoiding toxins, and getting enough sunlight and enough darkness at the right times. Best to turn that screen off before 8.00pm! Health is also about having enough leisure time and using it well; for meaningful, creative, soul-nourishing pursuits. (I'm not going to say "relaxation" because I don't want to sound like Emma's GP.)

More surprisingly, **your nutrition is not only about what food you eat**. Your nutritional status – how well nourished your body really is – also depends on at least nine other factors:

1 **When you eat.** Three meals a day still works well. Remember that pattern?! Three actual meals, no snacks in between. If you eat the meals, you won't need the snacks. Try not to skip breakfast, try not to forget lunch, and do remember to eat your evening meal sooner rather than later. Four hours before bedtime is ideal.

2 **Where you eat.** Not at your desk/on the bus/on the run! Sit down. Somewhere quiet and pleasant.

3 **How you eat.** Slowly. Take time to enjoy your food. Chewing thoroughly breaks food up into smaller pieces, so your digestive enzymes get more access to its surface. You'll digest it better, get more nutrients from it, and it will be longer before you get hungry again.

4 **Whether you are digesting properly.** Are your digestive enzymes working properly to break down your food? Is your stomach making enough acid? Is your liver making enough bile, and is the bile getting through to your small intestine? If you are eating right but feeling wrong, your digestion may need some attention – from a competent nutritional therapist, rather than the chemist! But equally, if you are under huge stress, your autonomic nervous system will be switched to "flight or fight" mode, as opposed to "rest and

digest" mode, so your digestion won't be able to work properly.

5 **Whether you are absorbing properly.** This is connected with your digestion, but is not the same. It means: are the digested, broken-down products of what you've eaten being absorbed from the gut into the bloodstream? This depends on the state of the epithelial cells that line the inner surface of your small intestine. Sometimes absorption can be very poor, as when the gut lining is damaged by an inflammatory condition such as Crohn's disease. But there are other instances where absorption is wrong in other ways; not necessarily the classic "malabsorption". For example, if you are not digesting (breaking down) food well, and you have a "leaky gut" (see page 84), you may be absorbing large molecules of food that ought not to get through into the bloodstream at all. If they do, they can trigger the immune system to react, and make you feel ill and groggy; this may be one of the mechanisms of food intolerance.

6 **How rapidly your body is using up the nutrients you are taking in.** If you are stressed and overworking, you use up your nutrients very fast, especially the B vitamins, Vitamin C and magnesium, as with Emma.

7 **Whether there are toxins in your system destroying the nutrients.** (More in Chapter 7.)

8 The state of your TTCs – Trillions of Tiny Companions.
These are the bacteria in your gut which are busy processing everything you swallow, for better or worse, according to what species of bugs are in there, and in what ratios. More about this in Chapter 2.

9 Where/when/how your food was grown/reared. Does it actually contain all the nutrients it is supposed to have? Which leads on to:

Do We Need Nutritional Supplements?

Well, we **shouldn't** need them, of course. Ideally, we'd get all our nutrients from food; that's the natural way. Before the Industrial Revolution, we could indeed have derived all the nutrients we needed from food. It was all grown locally and organically, and the time between picking and eating was minimal. Today, sadly, the famous "healthy balanced diet" is very hard to obtain, and here's why:

Our soil has been so depleted by intensive farming that the crops grown on it no longer contain the levels of minerals that they contained even 50 years ago.[32,33,34,35] The soil is as overworked as we are. Your average portion of broccoli, for example, is meant to contain plenty of magnesium. But it can only absorb magnesium through its root system if the magnesium is still there in the earth to be absorbed. Your broccoli has some magnesium, but you can be sure that it has much less than the same size portion in 1965. Similarly, Brazil nuts are supposed to be a rich source of selenium, but they won't be if the ground where the tree grows has been so over-farmed that it has become depleted of selenium. And so on.

Traditional farming involved rotating crops; because different plants absorb different minerals preferentially, the stubble was ploughed back in after harvesting, and each patch of land was allowed to lie fallow (growing no crops) every few years. The soil needs to rest from time to time, like we do. Also, traditional farmers had animals fertilising the ground naturally, whereas these days farm animals are kept separately from crops.

Furthermore, we now use fertilisers which force plants to grow faster, further depleting the soil. And the use of fungicides kills the mycorrhizae, beneficial fungi whose role is to "fix" nutrients from the soil into the roots of the plant. Therefore even such nutrients as do remain in the soil often do not find their way into our food crops. And farm animals are often fed on grain or grass that is similarly depleted, so our meat may be nutrient-deficient too, as well as being contaminated by herbicides.

Most of what we eat has been stored, transported, stored again and often processed, irradiated and packaged in plastic. It's no longer truly fresh, so it no longer contains sufficient levels of antioxidant nutrients. And there may be preservative gases in that plastic packaging along with your still-remarkably-fresh-looking salad.

For all these reasons, and also those listed in points 4–8 above, you may well need some nutritional supplements from time to time. Much more about this in subsequent chapters, especially Chapter 6, which tells you how to select supplements, and how to ensure that you are taking the right thing, at the right time, and nothing you don't actually need.

Your most important tool

At first, your most important tool for improving your health is – wait for it – **a magnifying glass**. No kidding. Especially if you're over 45, and struggling to read the small print on a long ingredients list. We must get wise to all the junk they're getting us to put into our bodies in the name of food.

Here's the ingredients list on a popular brand of "healthy yogurt", marketed at children:

Guar gum
Potassium sorbate
Maize starch
Concentrated apple juice (that's sugar)
Tri-calcium phosphate
Burnt sugar syrup (that's sugar)
Sodium citrate
Fructose (that's sugar)
Natural flavouring (But what is it?! I emailed and asked
    and got no reply)

All commercial "fruit yogurts", even the organic ones, have lots of sugar in, and very little fruit. If you want fruit yogurt, just mix some fruit into some plain yogurt! Remember, if it ends in "-ose", it's sugar. Glucose, dextrose, fructose, sucrose, maltose – it's all sugar. So is malto-dextrin. Don't buy it.

There are plenty of guidebooks to this hazardous territory: *E for additives, A–Z Guide to Food Additives, What's Really in your*

Basket? and more. Also *FIND OUT*, a little guide from Foresight, the pre-conception charity; Foresight is now sadly defunct, but you might get a copy on eBay. The guide is tiny, so it's very easy to take shopping.

One of these books says: "Never eat what you can't pronounce." They've got a point, but it might just be the Latin name of a plant, referring to a harmless and helpful herbal ingredient. So you need to get informed – and get that magnifying glass, because the most toxic stuff is printed really, really small.

Of course, real food doesn't come in a tin or a plastic package, and doesn't need an ingredients list. If you catch a fish or pick an apple, there's no ingredients list on it. Eventually, you'll ditch all the packaged stuff. But for now, you need that magnifying glass, and not just in the supermarket. You need it in the chemist; toiletries are full of toxic ingredients, and they do go into your body through your skin. You may even need it, sadly, in the health-food shop; that herbal shampoo may contain some herbal extracts, but it may contain some harsher chemicals too. And that "protein bar" is not protein, it's sugar. (Squashed dates are basically sugar.) Leave it in the shop – but if you are still craving it, ask yourself: did you skip lunch?

Don't be embarrassed to stand in the shop and read ingredients lists – you have a right to know what you are putting in or on your body. If a label says "free from artificial flavourings and colourings", don't take that at face value. Check it out, look and learn. You only have one body. And if you want to know more, beyond what's on the ingredients lists, check out two excellent and shocking books: *Not on the Label* by Felicity Lawrence, and *Swallow This* by Joanna Blythman.

And now, let's spring into Winter.

CHAPTER 1

WINTER

(December, January, February)

Winter is a time to withdraw a little, to wrap up warm and hunker down; in fact, to partially hibernate. It's a time to consolidate but not to start new projects, especially not ambitious plans like a weight-loss diet, which has a far better chance of success in the spring. In winter, nature is telling you to be indoors when it's dark, to be outside only in the limited hours of daylight, and generally to do less not more.

What's In Season And Good To Eat?

- **Root veg**. Tubers. Potatoes, sweet potatoes, pumpkin, parsnip, butternut squash, all other kinds of squash (the veg not the drink!), swedes, turnips and others. There are lots of fabulous recipes for these if you are bored with boring old boiling, although boiling does not ruin root veg nearly as much as it does greens. You can roast them in coconut oil, mash them with olive oil and spices, steam, braise, pressure-cook or slow-cook them, and they are cheap. This is not a recipe book, but all sorts of yummy recipes for root veg can be found everywhere from the BBC website to the plethora of new healthy cookbooks.

On the whole, it's better to get the majority of your carbohydrates from root veg rather than from grains. This is the evolutionary perspective again. The fact is, we have been digging up root veg and cooking them ever since we discovered fire a million years ago, whereas we have only been eating grains since we settled down and started farming a mere 10,000 years ago. Furthermore, wheat – the chief grain on which most of us are overdosing – is not what it once was. The wheat from which most bread sold in the UK is made has been selectively bred for over a century. It's a hybrid, with vastly more gluten in it than its wild ancestor contained. And that's quite apart from the dreadful additives put into most commercial bread these days. Get your magnifying glass out – our daily bread is bad news.

Winter greens. Cabbage, kale, chard, Brussels sprouts, cavolo nero (black kale), leeks, cauliflower, pak choi and so on. This is not the time for salads, or at least not often. This is the time for cooking. Greens should be lightly steamed, or sautéed; use coconut oil or butter, or chicken fat or lamb/beef/pork fat if you're not a vegetarian. But not vegetable oils – they turn into trans fats on heating to high temperatures.

Olive oil is ok for cooking at low temperatures. And make soup, using root veg and greens, onions and garlic and leeks, and meat or poultry.

⚘ **Meat and fish**. These are full of Vitamin D, which you absolutely need so your immune system can fight off all those winter infections. We can also make Vitamin D from the action of the sun on our skin; sunlight turns the cholesterol just under our skin into Vitamin D. BUT there is not remotely enough sunlight in a UK winter (or spring or autumn) to meet your body's need for Vitamin D. There just isn't – sorry! Meat should be free-range and organic, while fish should be sustainably caught, from clean waters. In the Arctic, people get their Vitamin D from fish. About salmon: be aware that all farmed salmon will have been bred in sea-cages. Unless it's organically farmed, it will also have been artificially coloured, and will not have had enough room to swim. Of course wild salmon is best, but it's not in season in winter. If the pack says "wild salmon" in January, it's either been frozen (which is fine) or it's a lie (which is not).

⚘ **Eggs**. These are full of good fats and proteins, most minerals and many vitamins. Easy to digest, quick to cook in the morning. Now let's be honest here; eggs are not strictly in season in winter; most birds start laying eggs in spring. So if you want to be a purist... but if you're not eating any meat or fish, then they really are vital in the winter. Please remember to make sure they are organic and free-range!

✑ **Nuts.** Preferably buy them in their shells, which naturally keep them fresh, and crack them open at home.

What Not To Eat In Winter? (At Least, Not Too Much)

✑ **Raw food**. People vary, of course, but most of us should be eating mostly cooked food in a British winter, and keeping the salads for summer. It's what your body tells you anyway, if you stop to listen. It's not rocket science, it's common sense. And if you're eating hot meals instead of salads, you might even find you can turn the central heating down a bit.

✑ **What about fruit?** Only citrus fruits could really be said to be in season in winter, and we gravitate towards them because we need the Vitamin C. If you stick to actual oranges/satsumas/grapefruits, not cartons of juice (too much sugar!) then it's ok from time to time. Of course they don't grow in the UK, so a purist would argue that it's not natural for us to be eating them – but life's too short to be a purist. Much more about fruit in the Autumn chapter. A word of caution about citrus fruits: they don't suit everyone. Best avoided if you are dealing with a duodenal or stomach ulcer. And some people with arthritis find that citrus worsens their condition.

✑ **What about apples and pears?** Well, they do keep if you wrap and store them properly, so I would extend autumn to

the end of December for this purpose. But they are better cooked than raw in cold weather, so stewed apples and baked pears are the order of the day, once or twice a week.

🌿 **Dairy produce**. Go easy on the dairy products in winter if you are prone to colds/coughs/sinus problems/earaches/ general snottiness. Dairy foods produce mucus, which can clog you up. Milk is not good for you anyway (see page 19).

Which Nutrients Do You Need Most In Winter?

Answer: Vitamin C, Vitamin D, Zinc, Selenium and Magnesium.

Vitamin C

Vital for the immune system to fight off those winter viral and bacterial infections. And didn't I just say the same thing about Vitamin D? I did indeed. You need both. But there's an important difference. Vitamin C is water-soluble; you use it up or pee it out within hours. So you need a daily supply; you can't store it. (Vitamin D, by contrast, is fat-soluble. This means you can store it in your body, so if – and it's a big if – you got enough of it from sunshine-on-the-skin during the summer, you may have stores that will last you through to the next summer. In practice this rarely works in the UK – unless you're a professional gardener – because there's not enough sun.)

Back to Vitamin C. It's in raw fruit and veg – and I've just said we shouldn't have too much of that in the winter. So where do we get it? Well, there is a little bit left in potatoes and root veg, even after cooking. There is some left in the pickled fruit and veg that our great-grandmothers made to see us through the winter, because they were always pickled in glass jars (it's the heat involved in putting food in tins that destroys all the Vitamin C). The best source is citrus fruit, but it's not enough. Remember, the Inuit peoples of the far north got their Vitamin C from the adrenal glands of the animals they ate, when they were still living in their traditional way. We probably did the same in a British winter in previous times; the adrenal gland sits on top of the kidney, and people certainly used to eat kidneys a lot more than they do now.

Also, crucially, our bodily requirement for Vitamin C is higher than it used to be. Stress, alcohol, cigarettes, pollution, even tea, coffee and Paracetamol – these things deplete us of Vitamin C, drain it out of the system. So we need more. We actually need a supplement, right through the winter, starting from a week or two before you usually go down with your first cold of the season – so hopefully you won't get that cold.

The majority of mammals can make their own Vitamin C, from glucose. But humans, guinea pigs and fruit bats can't; we need to eat some every day.

For most people I would recommend 500–1000 mg of Vitamin C, as ascorbic acid or magnesium ascorbate or potassium ascorbate, with each meal, from November through to March. Avoid the ascorbic acid version if you have duodenal or stomach ulcers; it is cheaper, but harsher on the gut lining. Don't get the effervescent version from the chemist – it's full of junk!

Vitamin C is also good at fighting cancer cells.[36,37,38] Our bodies produce cancer cells all the time, as random mutations, but an immune system in good condition will recognise them as "alien" and destroy them. The more we support the immune system, the better it will be at doing this vital job. There is good evidence for the role of Vitamin C, and other natural substances found in fruit and vegetables, in cancer prevention.[39]

Vitamin D

This has been mentioned already, as we need it so much, and so many of us are deficient. It's not only that it helps us fight infections. It also helps to prevent cancer, auto-immune disease, inflammatory conditions and mental illness, all of which are on the rise in the UK, and are noticeably rarer at the Equator. If you live in Britain and work indoors, you'll probably be Vitamin D-deficient by the end of the winter, and quite possibly even at the start of the winter. If you're vegan, that's not just probable, it's definite. And the darker your skin, the greater the risk.

Chapter 3 (Summer) will tell you how to maximise your production of Vitamin D from sunlight. Meanwhile, here's what to do in winter:

First, ask your GP to measure your Vitamin D level. It's a simple blood test. The result should be between 75 and 200 nmol/L (that's nano-mols per litre). That's what's called the Normal Range, and ideally you want your result to be somewhere in the middle of that range. But some GP surgeries have recently lowered their "Normal Range" to 50–150. That's plain wrong, and it's happened because of a confusion between what's **healthy** and what's **average**. They have found so many people's Vitamin D levels to be so much lower than expected, that instead of concluding that there's an epidemic of Vitamin D deficiency (there is), they have decided that their Normal Range must have been too high in the first place! (They've done the same goal-post shifting with thyroid hormone levels, by the way.) So if your Vitamin D level comes back at 50 nmol/L, you may be told it's borderline or satisfactory. It isn't. It's low.

Be careful about the units; most GP surgeries give Vitamin D results in nmols/L, as above, but some use µg/L (micrograms per litre), in which case the normal range that's equivalent to 75–200 nmol/L would be 30–80 µg/L.

Your GP learnt at medical school, as I did, that Vitamin D is needed for healthy bone development, and that without it children get rickets. This is true. But to get rickets (or the adult version, osteomalacia) your Vitamin D level would have to be very, very low; almost zero. We were **not** taught about all the other problems, mentioned above, that can result from sub-optimal Vitamin D levels. When I was at medical school, vitamins were mentioned once, in the only lecture in 6 years to cover nutrition. We were told that they were substances needed in tiny amounts to prevent specific "Deficiency Diseases". Thus a total lack of Vitamin D caused rickets, total lack of Vitamin C caused scurvy, total lack of Vitamin A caused blindness, total lack of Vitamin B1 caused Beri-beri, total lack of Vitamin B3 caused Pellagra, and total lack of Vitamin B12 caused Pernicious Anaemia. (Sadly, the quantity and quality of nutritional education for medical students hasn't improved much in the past 40 years; see page 254.)

This is all correct, but there was no understanding of the grey area, no concept of the vast and increasing territory that lies between complete health at one extreme and a specific, severe deficiency disease at the other. You can have vitamin deficiencies that are too mild to give you a recognised deficiency disease, too mild to kill you, but severe enough to make you tired and ill nevertheless.

Your GP may need a little persuading to do the Vitamin D blood test, as funds are tight. It sometimes helps if you mention your mother's and grandmother's osteoporosis. Here's the bone connection: Vitamin D ensures that calcium from your food is absorbed from the gut into the bloodstream. You do **not** need a calcium supplement – there's still enough calcium in food – you just need Vitamin D. Some GPs recommend a Vitamin-D-plus-calcium supplement; don't. Just take Vitamin D. Too much calcium pushes out magnesium, which your bones also need, and about which more below.

> **Which Vitamin D to take?**
> It must be Vitamin D3. That's what the sunlight makes in our skin. Beware of the cheap, ersatz version, Vitamin D2. It's synthetic junk, and it's counterproductive, but it's a common food additive as well as a bad supplement.

Vitamin D is found in all animal produce, particularly oily fish, i.e. salmon, mackerel, sardines, herring, trout, pilchards. There is no significant vegan source of Vitamin D3, except sunshine. Some vegan foods are artificially fortified with Vitamin D, but it's usually the junk version, D2; read the label and check!

Zinc

This is an important trace mineral, needed for the white blood cells of our immune system to do their many vital tasks, from fighting off winter flu bugs to healing up cuts and grazes. Zinc is also needed as a "co-factor" by a great number of the enzyme systems in the body, including our "Superoxide Dismutase" enzymes, whose job is to get rid of Superoxide, an example of a "free radical". "Free radicals" or "Reactive Oxygen Species" (ROS) are two clumsy names for waste products which we make naturally from energy-production metabolism in our cells. These waste products should get vacuumed up and destroyed instantly by our antioxidants, which include the Superoxide Dismutase enzymes themselves and also many specific nutrients such as zinc, selenium and vitamins A, C, E and B12. But this will only work if we've got enough of them.

Zinc is needed also for the functioning of an enzyme called Delta-6-Desaturase, which converts Essential Fatty Acids (EFAs) to their most useful, anti-inflammatory forms. If you're taking omega 3 or omega 6 EFAs for inflamed joints, they will work a whole lot better if you are taking zinc as well.

Insulin, a vital hormone for control of our blood sugar levels, requires zinc for its synthesis and storage in the pancreas. And we need zinc too for the senses of taste and smell.

Zinc is widely distributed in foods, both plant and animal foods. It is plentiful in nuts and seeds, grains and pulses, but as mentioned above, many people don't absorb zinc well from these sources, probably because plants contain phytates which prevent the absorption of zinc and other minerals. The richest source of zinc is oysters, but most of us rarely if ever eat oysters. So, you probably need a zinc supplement to get you through a British winter. See Chapter 6 for how to choose a good one.

Selenium

Also vital for the white blood cells of the immune system, as above, so selenium is part of your immune-boosting package to ward off flu and other infections. Selenium is also needed by the enzyme Glutathione Peroxidase, an important antioxidant. The best food source of selenium is Brazil nuts, but it is found in plenty of other foods too. When I do blood tests for selenium and zinc, I almost always find that zinc is deficient, whereas selenium is only sometimes low. This is important, because selenium is fairly easily absorbed, even by people with poor gut function, so there is a theoretical risk of overdosing if you were to take a selenium supplement all the year round.

I would recommend taking selenium only at those times of the year when you find yourself most likely to get ill with flu etc. That's winter for most people, but you know yourself best; it might be October or March. So take selenium only for 2–3 months a year, unless you can get your selenium level blood-tested by a nutritional therapist (see the Resources section), in which case you'll have an objective measure of what you need, and for how long.

Selenium is an anti-cancer nutrient, because of its supportive effect on the immune system, and prevention is better than cure. So do take some, but don't go over the dose suggested on the pot.

Magnesium

Incredibly important to our physical and mental health, and very many of us are deficient in it. Unlike zinc and selenium, magnesium is not a "trace" mineral, needed in tiny amounts. It is needed in large amounts, for our bones, our brains, our muscles, our blood vessels and our heart, and also for normal sleep, for the production of energy in the mitochondria (energy-generating organelles in our cells) and for the healthy functioning of every cell in the body.

Magnesium enables muscles to relax. Got tight shoulders? Backache? Sore leg muscles? Cramp at night? Physiotherapy and massage, osteopathy or chiropractic may help, but their benefits will be strictly temporary if your magnesium level is too low. Any muscle that a body-work therapist has coaxed into "letting go" will be contracted again within hours. Muscle action is a "Yin-Yang" affair; calcium enables muscles to contract, and magnesium enables them to stretch and relax. They work in tandem. But contrary to popular belief, most of us need more magnesium, *not* more calcium. And too much calcium can push magnesium out of the body, and clog the blood vessels of the heart.

The relaxing effect of magnesium on muscles applies not only to the voluntary, skeletal muscles that we use to move our bodies consciously. It applies also to the involuntary muscle that comprises the walls of hollow organs such as the womb, the bladder and the gut. Without sufficient magnesium, the womb, for example, cannot relax properly to release the menstrual flow. This is one of the causes of painful menstrual cramps, and magnesium is one of the remedies (see Chapter 5).

Among the hollow organs composed of involuntary muscle we have to include the blood vessels. When magnesium levels inside the muscle cells of the blood vessels are too low, over many years, those blood vessels will tighten up. They get stiffer, and the heart has to work harder to push the blood through them, around the body. So you can end up with cold peripheries and, more seriously, with high blood pressure, and therefore a worn-out, failing heart. I do not believe that restoring good magnesium levels can, by itself, **treat** high blood pressure or heart failure, but it may well have a role to play in preventing them (Chorus: Prevention is Better than Cure.)

Magnesium also plays a part in blood sugar stability, in brain function and in more than a hundred enzyme reactions in the body.

Why are so many people deficient in magnesium? Partly for the same reason we are deficient in other minerals; depletion of the soil, as mentioned earlier. But for two other reasons as well, specific to magnesium. Firstly, in some people, calcium supplements are to blame; calcium pushes magnesium out. Women of a certain age: you do **not** need those calcium pills to prevent osteoporosis. You need Vitamin D3, Vitamin K2 and lots of exercise; see Chapter 5.

Secondly, and this is crucial, psychological stress lowers our magnesium levels. We pee out excess magnesium when we are stressed. This is an evolutionary glitch of obscure origin; it must have served a purpose once, but now it's a liability, and we get into the vicious circle described in Emma's story on page 37: Stress → lose magnesium in urine → muscles tighten up → feel even more tense.

Our cave-dwelling ancestors would have experienced stress intensely but fleetingly; if they got away from the lion alive, they would have replenished their depleted magnesium fairly quickly by eating – guess what – green leafy veg. This is full of chlorophyll, which contains magnesium in its most natural form, most easily assimilated by the human gut.

Should you get your magnesium level checked by a blood test? Well, there's a problem here. God bless the NHS, but it mostly only measures "plasma magnesium" or "serum magnesium", i.e. how much magnesium is floating around dissolved in the bloodstream. That figure will almost always be normal; the body keeps up the level of plasma magnesium even when stores are running low, because the heart couldn't function otherwise. So that test won't tell you very much. What I've been talking about here, however, is the **intra-cellular** level of magnesium, i.e. how much magnesium there is **inside your cells**. That's a more accurate reflection of your body's level, as magnesium lives mostly inside our cells. It certainly can be measured by a blood test, although I doubt your GP will offer this. But it doesn't really matter: it is very difficult to overdose on magnesium.

For your mood, your muscles, your energy, the health of your heart and the whole of your body/mind, keep your magnesium level up. There are **three ways** to do this:

1 Sorry to shout but EAT YOUR GREENS. Mostly cooked; it's winter.

2 Put Epsom salts in your bath. Epsom salts are simply magnesium sulphate, and the magnesium goes in through your skin. More on how to do this in Chapter 7. If you don't have a bath tub, a little foot bath will help.

3 Consider taking a magnesium supplement. Make sure it's an
absorbable one though, not magnesium oxide, which just acts
as a laxative, going straight through you without raising your
magnesium level. More on this in Chapter 6 – it tells you
what to look for on the label.

Why magnesium in the winter particularly?

Well, magnesium is good for you all the year round. But here
are three reasons why I've put it in the Winter chapter:

First, winter is cold, which tends to make all our muscles
contract, including the small blood vessels of our hands and
feet. Some people get cramp. Others get blue/white numb
fingers and toes: Raynaud's Syndrome. Restoring a healthy level
of magnesium to the cells can help all this.

Secondly, some people get stressed and miserable in the winter.
Magnesium, along with Vitamin D, can help prevent and treat
this.

Thirdly, Winter is the first chapter, and magnesium is so very
important that I just couldn't wait until later in the book to tell
you about it!

Winter Case History: Young Thomas's Grumpiness

Thomas was a grumpy teenage boy when his mother first brought him to see me. She had brought him for four reasons: he was becoming depressed and sometimes aggressive, he was very tired and listless, he was off school much of the time with flu and he was under-performing at school. His teachers knew he was extremely bright and was not remotely reaching his potential. And he had exams coming up.

Breakfast for Thomas was either a croissant or nothing at all. A croissant is just nutritionless, quick-burning refined carbs, so either way his blood sugar would be too low by 10.30 in the morning to concentrate in class. At school lunch he again chose only carbohydrate, going for sweetcorn or mashed potato but without the accompanying meat or fish and veg. This is because his blood sugar was probably so low by then he naturally craved carbs to try and boost it – this is a very common vicious circle, and is why he would also finish his lunch with a bar of chocolate.

Eating dinner at home was a strain; his mother offered him a proper meal, but he only wanted pizza or pasta. He would eat some meat but only "junk" meat: burgers, sausages and so on. He wouldn't touch fish or eggs or fruit or veg, except for pickled cucumber.

Thomas was also playing on his phone till midnight every night. Most screens emit a blue light, or a bright white light that contains blue light. It's the colour of the daytime sky. It tells the pineal gland in our brain that it is morning, time to be awake. That is one of the reasons that it is hard to sleep properly after staring at the screen (TV or computer or phone) all evening.

By midnight, Thomas had been staring at screens for so long that his pineal gland had not produced enough melatonin to let him fall asleep. The pineal gland can only produce melatonin, the sleep hormone, in darkness. Screen-light jinxes it. Therefore he couldn't sleep. So he turned the phone on again, trying to entertain himself, because he was bored and miserable as well as tired – another vicious circle.

We did blood tests for nutrient levels. Not surprisingly, Thomas turned out to have very low levels of Vitamin D and magnesium, and desperately low zinc. He was also very low in iodine, a vital nutrient that we haven't mentioned yet, found mostly in fish and seaweed, neither of which Thomas ate.

Confronted with the evidence, the numbers in front of him, Thomas said he was prepared to change his diet. But only a bit, because he still hated the taste and texture of vegetables, fish and eggs. Furthermore, Thomas couldn't swallow capsules, so I found him liquid versions of the supplements he needed. He took drops of Vitamin D, zinc and iodine in water. But he couldn't handle the taste of the liquid magnesium. So instead he agreed to do an Epsom salts bath every evening, allowing the magnesium to soak in through his skin. This had the added benefit of being an alternative to screen time; his parents fitted a dimmer switch outside the bathroom, and turned the lights low, and Thomas listened to music in the bath instead of staring at a screen. After two or three months he started sleeping better, and getting out of bed in the morning with less drama.

I also gave Thomas a lot of Vitamin C (as magnesium ascorbate powder dissolved in water), mixed with the other liquid supplements. I wanted to give Thomas a B-vitamin complex as well, to boost his energy and brain function, but he couldn't stand the taste of the liquid version, even in orange juice, although that works well for most children and teens. So that had to wait.

Three months later, Thomas was somewhat more alert and cheerful, and doing a bit better at school. That was due to improved sleep (thanks to the magnesium baths and a bit less screen-time) and to the iodine and Vitamin D, both of which improve brain function considerably. He had also started eating eggs, real meat, broccoli and tomatoes spontaneously. This is because zinc tunes up the taste buds, so people start actually **wanting** the food they **need**.

Another three months on, Thomas was achieving substantially better at school – he got excellent GCSE results – and was far pleasanter to live with. He described himself as no longer depressed. BUT it was now high summer. He was playing tennis, his exams were over; of course he felt better. The real test would be the following winter.

In September we repeated all Thomas's blood tests; iodine and zinc had normalised, while magnesium and Vitamin D had nearly normalised. Interestingly, Thomas said he could now no longer stand the taste of the zinc drops. This is the "zinc taste test" and was a good sign. When a person is zinc-deficient, their taste buds don't work properly, so they don't taste the zinc drops (or anything else) properly. Once the body's zinc level is corrected, the zinc drops begin to taste revolting. So it's time to stop them. Thomas's experience agreed with the repeat blood test result.

Thomas started double maths and physics A levels. He agreed to turn off all screens – computer, phone and TV – by 9.00pm, a degree of cooperation that would have been unthinkable a few months earlier. He also decided that he would try to swallow a capsule, so he could take the Vitamin B complex at breakfast to boost his energy and brainpower. He managed this about five mornings out of seven, which was fine.

When November came, Thomas made sure he was taking plenty of Vitamin C at every meal, and at the first sign of a cold he would add in some zinc, selenium and echinacea (a herb that supports the immune system). He got one mild cold that winter, at the start of the Christmas holidays, but that was all. He didn't get the flu.

By the spring, 15 months after his first consultation, Thomas was off all supplements and doing well. He was calm and balanced, had plenty of energy, and was doing fine in his studies. What he needs to remember in winter, as well as his vitamins C and D, is to get some outdoors time in the daylight hours. He still needs reminding about that. But he does now remember to have break- fast every day, and he eats a lot more real food, although he'll always be a fussy eater.

Thomas would still prefer the system that some American high schools have, whereby the school day runs from 11.00am to 5.00pm, rather than 9 to 3. It suits teenagers' natural rhythms better. Nevertheless, he's managing to get to school on time most days, even in a UK winter. And he now understands the addictive power of electronic screens, and how destructive that can be to his mental health. He rations his own screen time, because he knows he feels better when he limits it. And he wants to do well at university, where he won't have his mum in the next room to remind him: "Time to switch off, now, Thomas!"

Health Hazards Of Winter And How To Prevent Them

I will mention five of these; the first three are closely related.

1 Hibernation failure
2 SAD
3 Infections
4 Raynaud's Syndrome
5 Indoor pollution

Hibernation failure

Winter is naturally a time to hibernate (Latin *hibernus* = winter). Not completely, like a bear or a tortoise, but partially, like a natural human. So the first hazard is what I would call "Hibernation Failure" – trying to live as fully and energetically and "out there" as if it were summer, and the days were long.

If we have a choice, we need to do less of everything in the winter. Be at home more, out and about less. Winter is **not** a time to start new projects. And January 1st might just be the worst possible time to make a resolution; energy and willpower are at their lowest. The Persians have the Spring Equinox (March 21st) as their New Year, and the early Romans had March 1st; those make more sense. Plants are dormant in the winter, and so are many animals. We too are animals, there's no getting away from it.

Winter is therefore not the time to begin, for example, a weight-loss diet. It's cold, and the body wants to store fat for insulation. Wait till spring; you'll have more energy, feel more inclined to exercise, and find it much easier to eat less. So you're more likely to succeed.

Seasonal Affective Disorder (SAD)

This just means feeling miserable in winter. It's often partly down to Vitamin D deficiency, but only partly. Whatever our Vitamin D level, we do need to get some daylight in winter, to avoid SAD. In midwinter that's only possible between 8.00am and 4.00pm in the south of England, and between 9.00am and 3.00pm in the north of Scotland. The good news is that even with total cloud cover, some sunlight is getting through, otherwise it would be totally dark. And your pineal gland needs that daylight. (Descartes thought the pineal was the seat of the soul; modern endocrinology textbooks barely mention it.) So walk outdoors in the daylight. But other than that, apart from essentials like work and shopping, take it easy.

Infections

Most of us, of course, don't have much choice. We have to get up for work just as early in winter as in summer. We often leave the house in the dark and come home in the dark. We're fighting our biology at every step, and it takes its toll. That's why we get ill, that's why we come down with flu. So here's a prevention and **first-aid package** to keep in your kitchen from October to March, though you'll need it most in December and January. This is adapted from the work of my colleague Dr Sarah Myhill, and you can find a fuller version on her brilliant website, drmyhill.co.uk. Here's my version:

- Vitamin C: 500–1000 mg at every meal
- Zinc: 15 mg daily
- Selenium: 100 µg daily
- Echinacea: 15 drops 2 or 3 times daily

(See Chapter 6 for details of how to choose supplements.)

This is all to boost your immune system, which is low in winter but lower still when we have to go against our instincts and behave as though it wasn't winter at all. This "first-aid package" – Dr Myhill's version includes Vitamins A and E, and propolis too – is both prevention and treatment. If you take it daily through the winter, it should prevent flu and colds, provided you also get enough sleep. But if you feel yourself coming down with a bug, or if someone else in your household is getting ill, you can double all the above dosages until it's passed off. Even if you do still catch a cold, the first-aid package should make it briefer and much milder.

Raynaud's Syndrome

Also known as Raynaud's Phenomenon or Raynaud's Disease, it's a common hazard in a British winter. The fingers and/or toes go cold, numb, white, yellow or blue, when the weather's even slightly cold. If you are prone to this, and you can't move to somewhere nice and warm, then you need to maximise your magnesium intake, as outlined above. Magnesium will relax the smooth muscle of the small blood vessels, encouraging them to open up and maintain better circulation to your peripheries. Vitamin E helps too, as do Essential Fatty Acids, both fish oils (omega 3) and evening primrose oil (omega 6). Exercise helps the blood vessels open up; caffeine and cigarette smoke shut them down.

Indoor pollution

Our homes are full of chemicals we know nothing about. From the fire-retardants in our curtains to the air-freshener in our loo, from the insecticide in our carpet to the chlorine in our disinfectant. From the synthetic perfume in our laundry powder to the stain-remover we just sprayed on the sofa; all these and many more are toxic to living cells. They are there all the year round, and more about how to survive/avoid them in Chapter 7, but **in winter they build up because we don't open the windows**.

Take-Home Tips For Winter

 Eat more cooked than raw food. Soups. Casseroles.

 Take Vitamin C, zinc and a little selenium at breakfast. Take Vitamin D and magnesium at dinner.

 Ask your GP to keep an eye on your Vitamin D level – but avoid taking Vitamin D supplements in the 48 hours before the blood test.

 Go for a walk outdoors during the brief hours of daylight – best way to avoid getting SAD.

🌿 Keep the "first-aid package" (see page 67–68) handy from October to March. If you're not taking it routinely, start it at the first sign of a sniffle. Your own sniffle or that of anyone with whom you share a house or office!

🌿 Limit screen time for yourself and your children. Develop the habit of switching off a few hours before bedtime. (Actually this applies all the year round.)

🌿 Don't buy new mattresses, curtains, carpets or sofas in the depths of winter. They out-gas toxins; see Chapter 7. Wait till spring, and then keep the windows open.

🌿 Don't start new projects in winter. When possible, have a totally guilt-free duvet day at the weekend. Hibernate.

CHAPTER 2
SPRING

(March, April, May)

The sap is rising, the mornings are lighter; come out of hibernation and start afresh! Get up in time to have a proper breakfast – you'll have a better day. If you need to build up your level of exercise, and/or to lose weight, spring is the right season to begin those projects. If you find that the exercise is wearing you out, or that the weight is not coming off even though you're doing everything right, ask your GP to check your thyroid hormone level.

What's In Season And Good To Eat?

Remember, spring weather is unpredictable, so eat according to the actual temperature, not the calendar!

- **Spring greens, spring onions, rocket, radish, rhubarb.**
  Also some kale, chard, leeks and root vegetables still going from last year. In late spring, new season spinach and

purple-sprouting broccoli. Veg growers call late spring the HUNGRY GAP. A good way to fill this gap is by sprouting seeds and growing salad leaves on your windowsill. It's very easy: see page 76.

🌿 **Eggs**

🌿 **Dairy products.** But not if you suffer from asthma, eczema, hayfever or sinus problems.

🌿 **Spring lamb.** Don't assume that all sheep live their whole lives grazing freely on the hillsides and fields; most do, but not all. Make sure that what you are buying is genuinely free-range, as well as organically reared.

What's Out Of Season?

🌿 **Fruit!** With one exception – rhubarb. Cook rhubarb with honey, but gradually reduce the amount of honey you use; see how low you can go. Spring is a good time to retrain your taste buds. Add cinnamon/nutmeg/ginger or whichever spices you fancy.

Which Nutrients Might You Be Lacking?

After a long winter, you might be low in **Vitamin C**, **Vitamin D**, and the minerals **zinc**, **magnesium**, **selenium** and **iodine**, i.e. all the nutrients mentioned in the last chapter, if you weren't supple-menting them through the winter. And if you found winter a stressful/depressing time, you may well be lacking the B vitamins now.

Vitamin C and the **B vitamins** are water-soluble; you just pee out whatever is surplus to the requirements of the moment. This means there is no risk of overdosing, so it is safe and sensible to take some. (See Chapter 6 for how to select junk-free, effective versions.) Regarding **Vitamin D**, ask your GP to measure your level if that didn't happen during the winter, and remember you are aiming for the normal range described on page 53. Don't accept a receptionist telling you on the phone that it's "ok" or "borderline"; you need a print-out with numbers and units on it! If it's below the normal range, as it will be if you weren't taking it through the UK winter, then you should take a Vitamin D3 supplement at least until May. Chapter 6 gives suggested dosages based on the test results you get from your GP.

For the functions of Vitamins C and D in the body, see the previous (Winter) chapter. The B vitamins assist with energy production, sugar metabolism, detoxification and many other func-tions, and they help with alertness and mental clarity too. Best taken at breakfast, not dinner. There are lots of them, all with different but overlapping roles, and they all work together and help each other. That's why it's usually best to take a "B" complex, which contains all of them.

A Vitamin B complex caveat

There is a tiny minority of people who cannot cope with one or more of the B vitamins, except in minuscule doses. This is very rare, but if you do have a bad reaction, such as a headache, to taking a B complex, first check that it is a junk-free version, and you're not just reacting to an artificial additive. Once that's established, you have two options: (1) try a liquid version, and if the bottle says "10 drops daily" then start with just ONE drop daily, in a glass of water, sipped slowly in the morning. Build up the dose over several days, but not beyond what feels comfortable; you may not get up to the full recommended dose. That's ok. Option (2) is to consult a nutritional therapist, who can work out which of the B vitamins you are lacking, and which you may be genetically sensitive to. She/he can help you with trying out each of the B vitamins separately, on a "suck it and see" basis. To reiterate, this problem applies to very few people.

Minerals: **zinc** is needed for the reasons described in the Winter chapter, and most people's immune systems will benefit from continuing to take zinc up till April. With **selenium**, however, you should be more cautious. Again, it supports the immune system to ward off coughs and colds and cancer,[40,41] but if you took it for 2–3 months of the winter that's probably enough till next November/December. If you didn't, then take some now, for 2–3 months. Then stop. You can then keep the level up by eating Brazil nuts. **Magnesium** – this is beneficial all the year round, especially if you are stressed or suffering from stiff, tense muscles. More detail on magnesium can be found on pages 57–61.

Iodine is vital for all the body's cells, not just for the thyroid gland. It is particularly important to keep breast tissue healthy, and there is some evidence for its role in prevention of breast cancer.[42,43] It occurs in the sea, from which we evolved, and it occurs in the soil, but far less reliably. Most of us are not getting enough. Fish, seafood and seaweed are the only significant food sources of iodine, so vegetarians and vegans should ensure they incorporate some seaweed into their diet. Dried strips of wakame, nori, kombu or dulse are great in soups, stews and casseroles, and can be bought in most health-food shops or Japanese supermarkets.

There is an important reason why many of us are deficient in iodine, and it's not just about diet. The elements fluorine, chlorine and bromine are common environmental pollutants now, and they push iodine out of the body, possibly replacing it in the tissues where it should be. Conversely, if we start off with low iodine levels, those contaminants are more able to get into our bodies. Fluorine in the form of fluoride is in most toothpaste and many mouthwashes, chlorine is in our tap water as an antibacterial, and bromine is in the fire retardants which are put into all synthetic soft furnishings. (More about this in Chapter 7.) You can protect yourself somewhat by taking iodine in the form of a capsule of kelp (seaweed) every day.

The benefits of iodine have been known for centuries, and are part of the medical wisdom that has been lost in the Age of Drugs. Even now, though, iodine is still used in operating theatres as a safe and powerful antiseptic/disinfectant. And in the form of iodide it has numerous uses; this knowledge was still current when I was a medical student in the late 70s and early 80s. The saying was, with regard to any illness that was hard to diagnose and hard to treat:

"If you know not what or why, give the patient K and I."

K means potassium, I means iodide. KI, potassium iodide, was the "go-to" remedy for "difficult cases".

As well as lacking specific vitamins and minerals in spring, you may be lacking any of the numerous compounds found in plants, which enhance our health in ways we are only just beginning to recognise. These substances are known collectively as "**phytonutrients**" – "phyto" is Greek for plant – and it seems there's a new one popping up every minute. The best way to get those phytonutrients in spring is to **sprout your own salad** on your windowsill. You do need some raw veg now, but what's in the shops has been shipped from far-away polytunnels and is neither fresh nor cheap. Furthermore, tiny young plants are far more digestible than larger, older ones, so you'll get more nutritional mileage out of growing your own.

Sprouting your own salad

Many seeds sprout well on a window ledge: mung beans are the easiest, but you can try lots of others, such as alfalfa, broccoli, aduki beans, sunflower seeds, chickpeas and so on. Sprouted mung beans are the "bean shoots" you get in Chinese restaurants, but yours will be greener because they won't be deprived of light. You can use a jar, or get a sprouter from a hardware shop, health-food shop or online. It's just a set of three or four small, square trays made of hard, see-through plastic, that stack on top of one another. All the trays have holes in except the bottom one, which catches the drips when you water your seedlings. You should rinse and then pre-soak the seeds in water overnight, and – here's the nutritional trick – add liquid minerals to the water you soak the seeds in. So a few drops of liquid zinc, selenium if you need it, chromium if you have blood sugar issues, or whatever you need. The seeds will absorb the minerals and incorporate them into the little shoots in a far more absorbable, natural form than you get in any tablet or capsule.

Once they've been soaked for about 12 hours, spread the seeds out on the sprouting trays; not too many at once, or they'll crowd each other. Leave them on a ledge or worktop near a window, and water once or twice a day. Ideally, filter your tap water (see Chapter 7) so you are not watering your seedlings with chlorinated water; they'll absorb the chlorine and it's bad for you. Different seeds sprout at different rates, but most are ready in a few days.

Sprouted broccoli seedlings are slightly spicy, and even more nutritious than mature broccoli. The 3-day-old seedlings contain vastly more Di-Indolyl Methane (DIM) and Sulphoraphane weight-for-weight than does mature broccoli. These substances help convert oestrogen into its safer (non-carcinogenic) form in the body. This means that potentially broccoli sprouts eaten regularly could be protective against the commoner types of breast cancer. But a word of warning – when they start sprouting, they first grow hundreds of tiny, white, root hairs. Some people mistakenly think this is mould, and throw them away. It isn't, so don't! Have a look through your magnifying glass and you'll see. You can get a packet of A. Vogel's

"BioSnacky" Broccoli Rapini seeds from the Natural Dispensary.

Eat your sprouted seedlings with anything and everything. If you put them in a stir-fry, do so at the very last minute, so they're warm but still essentially raw; that conserves all those phytonutrients and antioxidants, which fight "free radicals" and reduce inflammation.

Growing actual salad leaves like lettuce can also be done on your windowsill, but you'll need a window box or some small pots full of organic soil or compost. Again, don't wait till they are full size; pick and eat them little. They are tastier and more nutritious when they're small. And there's something in between mini-plants and sprouted seedlings, known as microgreens; also well worth checking out.

Health Hazards Of Spring And How To Prevent Them

Hay fever
This is dealt with in depth in the case history on page 92.

Weed-killer and other Biocides
Be aware: your local council may be, unwisely, using its last remaining pennies to spray weed-killers such as glyphosate ("Round-up") on parks and grass verges near your home. The guys doing it will usually be wearing protective gear, but you won't

when you turn up the next day with your toddler for a game of ball or an early picnic on the grass. Weed-killers (herbicides) are toxic to plants (except grass, which can survive almost anything) and they are toxic to us too.[44] Any chemical that damages living things will likely damage other living things; we do share most of our genes and biochemical processes with weeds, trees, butterflies and bears.

This spraying happens in summer too, but I'm mentioning it now because many councils start in spring. Ask them whether and when they are doing it! Finding out may involve a fight with their Kafkaesque bureaucracy, but you need to know. If the council can't or won't tell you, contact PAN, the Pesticide Action Network. They have successfully persuaded several towns in the UK to stop using glyphosate, and their "Pesticide-free Towns" campaign continues.

If you live in the countryside, the risk is of local (non-organic) farmers spraying their fields and orchards with similar "-cide" chemicals: pesticides, insecticides, fungicides, herbicides – they all kill living beings, and their collective name is "Biocides". "Bios" means life in Greek and "cida" means killer in Latin. Again, ask the farmers when and where they plan to spray. Ideally, go away for a few days, leaving your windows tight shut. I have seen many rural dwellers become seriously ill, mostly with neurological diseases, when the prevailing wind has blown these biocides towards their house. These chemicals damage our brain and nervous system most. Some farmers have died from the effects of these biocides.[45]

There are two other important sources of insecticide poisoning that you may not have thought of. The flea collar you put on your dog or cat is impregnated with insecticides; ditto if you put drops between your pet's shoulder blades. And when you rub that stuff from the chemist into your child's hair to get rid of nits – that's insecticide too, and it goes into the bloodstream through the skin of the scalp. These substances are poisonous. But there are some totally safe alternatives, for cats and dogs and children, and I describe them in detail in Chapter 3, because although nits and pet fleas can occur in spring (or at any time of year) they are an even bigger problem in summer.

Spring cleaning

I'm going to make a radical suggestion here. I'm going to suggest that if you want to do some spring cleaning, you SPRING CLEAN YOUR GUT NOT YOUR HOUSE. I will explain what I mean, why and how to do it below, but first let me explain why I've listed "spring cleaning" as a HAZARD.

The chemicals that most of us use for cleaning our houses are toxic. Try doing a quick inventory of the bottles stashed under your kitchen sink. Detergents, disinfectants, carpet cleaner, washing-up liquid, furniture polish – all of them. Check the bathroom too. Now have a look at their ingredients – they're listed on the bottle, but you may need your magnifying glass again. Sometimes you will even see the skull and cross-bones sign on there. We've become a bit desensitised to this sign, but it means what it has always meant: danger. For every one of these chemicals there is a Data Sheet, freely available, and you can look it up. What you'll see, though, is the effects of **acute** exposure, i.e. accidental splashing of the skin or eyes with these chemicals, or accidental ingestion. What is not shown is the effect of thousands of low-dose exposures accumulating over time, i.e. **chronic** exposure. We absorb these chemicals, partly through the skin but mostly through our lungs – we breathe them in. This inhalation of cleaning chemicals is much worse with aerosol sprays than with cream cleaners. And of course it's also worse with the windows shut.

There are plenty of harmless substances you can use instead, such as vinegar, and there is lots of excellent information on how to do this in the book *Cleaning Yourself to Death* by Pat Thomas.

Safe spring cleaning of your house begins with identifying the toxins in your cupboards and learning to avoid them. And perhaps we should question what we mean by "clean"? The chemical industry would like us to think that a really clean home environment is one from which every microorganism, every last bacterium, has been removed. Yet such an environment is dead, sterile and unnatural. It belongs only in the operating theatre. We evolved with billions of bacteria around us, on us and inside us. It is counter-productive (and actually impossible) to get rid of them all. So ditch the antibacterial spray, the antibacterial gel and the antibacterial wipes. Water and soap will usually do fine – preferably a safe, natural, chemical-free soap.

Cleaning and allergies

There is mounting evidence that our increasing obsession with hygiene has made our kids more vulnerable to allergies of all sorts. This comes as no surprise: if we remove every speck of dirt, we remove the immune system's training ground. Do you insist that the kids wash their hands when they come in from playing in the park or garden? This is a tricky one. I would say that if you can be sure that they've had no contact with dog or cat poo or weed-killer, then you don't need to insist. Otherwise, yes, but soap and water will do fine. Travelling in the car or on public transport makes you far dirtier than the park or garden does. That's toxic dirt.

Why Spring Clean Your Gut?

It's highly likely that what's inside you needs a spring clean rather more urgently than what's around you in your house. Remember I mentioned our TTCs – Trillions of Tiny Companions? I'm referring to what is now called the microbiome, or the microbiota; the literally trillions of microorganisms that make their home in our large intestine (colon).

There is a huge diversity of species in there – or there should be – and although each of these bugs is microscopically tiny, there are so many of them that their total weight adds up to 1 or 2 kg! They are now considered to constitute an actual organ of the body. We live in symbiotic relationship with them (Greek: sym = together, bios = life); they couldn't live without us, and we can't live without them either. They're also known as Commensals, from the Latin: mensa = table, com = with. They're with us at our table. Here's the reason I've called them "Companions". A companion means "one with whom you share bread" (Latin: com = with, pan = bread). Oh boy, do they share our bread! Whatever we eat, they eat. Altering your diet radically and quite quickly alters the ratios of the different types of TTCs in your gut.

Why on earth do they need spring cleaning? Well, inside many of us today in the "developed" world, the microbiome has become profoundly unbalanced. The numbers and ratios of the different species of these creatures has gone way out of kilter. For example, there should be thousands of species of bacteria (both aerobic and anaerobic species), and just a very few yeasts (single-celled fungal organisms). But again and again, stool tests (ordered by myself and my colleagues) are showing an excess of the yeasts, including weird ones that shouldn't be there at all, and of unfriendly bacteria as well. They also show a startling **lack** of many of the most friendly, helpful bacteria that we need in large amounts.

The friendly bacteria will make substances our bodies need (so long as we eat our greens!) such as vitamin K and some B vitamins like Biotin. The unfriendly ones release toxic waste products that can make us feel ill or tired, or cause "brain fog".

This imbalance, the decrease in the good TTCs and the increase in the "hostile" ones, is called **dysbiosis**. When, as is often the case, it is specifically an increase in yeasts or fungi, it can be called Fungal-Type Dysbiosis or FTD. This type of dysbiosis was first described in a medical journal back in 1931 by Hurst and Knott.[46] It was described again in 1964 by Winner and Hurley,[47] and again in 1978[48] and 1984[49] by Dr Orian Truss. In 1986 Dr William Crook wrote a book about it called *The Yeast Connection*,[50] and there have been numerous scholarly articles since those days, including by Drs John Howard, Adrian Hunnisett, Stephen Davies[51] and Leo Galland.[52] Dr Keith Eaton and others published several research articles about it between 2000 and 2004.[53,54,55]

Nevertheless, the mainstream of the medical profession has been very slow to accept the reality of what is going on in the human gut. As recently as 2014 many gastroenterologists were still, if you'll pardon the pun, pooh-poohing the whole concept of dysbiosis, and indeed until a couple of years ago, if I mentioned the state of a patient's microbiome (TTCs) in a letter to their GP, the response was ridicule or silence. And one of my patients was told by a gastroenterologist quite recently that what he ate would "make no difference" to the state of his gut.

The "Candida Hypothesis" was considered to be in the realm of "Alternative Medicine", even though all the authors mentioned above were/are professional doctors. Part of the problem was that Candida tended to die on the way to the lab, so it was hard to grow in stool cultures. Techniques of microbiology are better now, so we find it more often. We may also be finding it more often because so many people's guts have such an excess of it. And Candida is not the only fungus among us; there are many more types, all of them over-growing.

One of the ways that fungal organisms like Candida may do damage is that they can change from a yeast form to a "mycelial" form, in which they send out filaments (known as hyphae) which can penetrate the gut lining, loosening what should be "tight junctions" between adjacent cells. This leads to "**leaky gut**", another concept scornfully dismissed until recently, but now more and more accepted as it comes to be known by the more scientific-sounding name of "Intestinal Hyperpermeability". As Dr Michael Mosley says: "There is now clear evidence that leaky gut, or 'intestinal hyperpermeability', is a real condition".[56]

Why does leaky gut matter? Because our food is meant to be absorbed into the bloodstream only when it has been thoroughly broken down into its very small constituent molecules. If Candida

& Co have punched holes in the gut lining, then peptides – chunks of incompletely digested protein, too large to get through a healthy gut lining – will find their way through the gaps and into the bloodstream. This is a problem, because they may mimic hormones or neurotransmitters and produce all sorts of weird symptoms. Or, more commonly, they may trigger the immune system to produce antibodies against them, as it would to bits of alien protein from bacteria. Hence the reactions that we know as **food intolerance** and possibly autoimmunity as well.[57]

SIBO (Small Intestinal Bacterial Overgrowth), is a similar problem, which my colleagues in the BSEM have also been diagnosing and treating since the 1990s; equally, till recently, ignored or denied by the profession at large. So it is very heartening to see medicine at last catching up with our runaway TTCs; a rash of popular new books by expert doctors attests to the fact that what was once "wacky" or "quacky" is now mainstream. And so it goes.

Gut dysbiosis (whether FTD or SIBO) is strongly associated with IBS (Irritable Bowel Syndrome) which was previously considered to be primarily a psychological condition. Even today, people with IBS symptoms are more often offered counselling or anti-depressants than a stool test and probiotics (friendly bacteria in a capsule – more anon). Of course, IBS, like most illnesses, can be exacerbated by emotional distress, and a trauma can spark off an episode of it. But the root cause is in the gut, and IBS, unknown before the Industrial Revolution, has become more common in recent decades because the underlying condition, gut dysbiosis, has become more common.

Recent thinking is that even the more serious gut diseases such as Crohn's disease and ulcerative colitis (collectively known as inflammatory bowel disease or IBD) may be associated with severe gut dysbiosis. Certainly the gut is leaky in Crohn's disease.[58] But the effects of dysbiosis reach far beyond the gut, affecting the brain and the rest of the body too. Imbalance of our TTCs has been linked to obesity, diabetes, heart disease and more.

There are many causes of fungal type dysbiosis or FTD, and most of them probably apply to SIBO too; the single most important one is **too much sugar** in our diet. Sugar feeds yeast, as you know if you have ever baked your own bread. Adding even a small quantity of sugar to the mix causes the yeast to reproduce at a great rate, multiplying itself and releasing gases in the process. These gases are what causes the bread to rise; that's what the bubbles or air spaces are in bread. But those same sorts of gases will equally be released by the yeasts in your gut every time you feed them sugar! Cakes, biscuits, ice cream, sweets – whatever the source of the sugar, the yeasts in your gut think it's Christmas, and they celebrate, reproducing like crazy and making the gases that, in the mildest cases, cause embarrassing amounts of wind and in the worst cases cause abdominal cramps, bloating and an "airlock" in the gut past which nothing is flowing freely, leading to diarrhoea and constipation (yes, both) and a lot of pain and discomfort. (For tips on breaking the sugar habit, see pages 24–26.)

In addition to overdoing the sugar, there are other factors contributing to the epidemic of gut dysbiosis. **Antibiotics**, still given out far too casually, kill many gut bugs, good and bad alike. But the bad ones develop resistance and overgrow, leaving us with a deficit of some really essential TTCs. And remember, antibiotics don't just come from the GP. If you're not eating organic, you are eating antibiotics with your meat, eggs, dairy produce and even non-organically-farmed fish.

The contraceptive pill is also a factor, as higher levels of oestrogen and progesterone favour the overgrowth of fungal organisms. This occurs in pregnancy, of course, which is why thrush is common then. (Thrush is a vaginal infection with the yeast Candida albicans.) But pregnancies only last nine months, and women often take the pill for many years.

We must also mention **stress**, as it weakens the immune system (much of which lives in the gut), rendering it less able to fight off unfriendly organisms. Stress has this effect partly by raising our level of the hormone cortisol (taking steroid drugs has the same yeast-promoting effect).

I find the best way to understand gut dysbiosis is to compare the gut to a piece of land. Whether it's in a wood or a field, there should be lots of plants and animals flourishing there; there should be biodiversity. On a small-scale, old-fashioned organic farm, there will still be this biodiversity, with multiple species living co-operatively together. Then along comes agribusiness with its insecticides and herbicides, and kills three-quarters of the species living there. What will happen? The few species which can survive those biocides – the resistant ones – will now have the field to themselves; they will grow like mad and take over.

This leads to "monocrop" farming, and is quite deliberate. Any creature which feeds on those few surviving plants will have a field day eating them all up, so the farmer will need to use a pesticide against that creature – and so on forever, in a toxic cascade. This is roughly analogous to what happens in our gut when we take too many antibiotics. You can see there's a direct parallel between what's happening to the planet and what's happening in our intestines: decreasing biodiversity, species loss and increasing toxicity.

Again, if "Big Ag" comes along with a bag of artificial fertiliser, that causes certain species to grow too fast, depleting the soil of its vital nutrients in the process. Similarly, when we eat sugar, we're feeding the wrong creatures too much and too fast, and we can also become nutrient-depleted as a result. Sugar is an "anti-nutrient", and the worst kind of "fertiliser", over-feeding all the wrong bugs.

How To Spring Clean Your Gut

1 **Do it slowly and gently.** Do NOT rush off and try one of the "colon cleanse" or "liver cleanse" fads advertised on the internet. They can be dangerous, and even if they don't harm you, any benefits will be strictly temporary.

2 **Check out how much sugar you are eating.** Remember, milk contains sugar, and any ingredient ending with the suffix "-ose" is a sugar. Reduce your sugar intake over a couple of weeks, so that it gets to more or less zero. Replace the sugar in your diet with real foods, especially vegetables. If you are thin, you must also replace the sugar with healthy fats, such as avocado, nuts, seeds, coconut oil and olive oil. Remind yourself of the first two golden rules on pages 22–26.

You need lots of plant fibre to feed the healthy microbiota. Dr Denis Burkitt (1911–1993) noted in the 1950s and 60s that

African people eating their traditional diet did not develop colon cancer or many other Western diseases.[59] He understood that this was due to the high level of fibre in their diet (and also to the squatting as opposed to sitting position used for opening the bowels), but he thought that plant fibre simply assisted the gut motility. It certainly does do that, but now we know that it is also essential food for our TTCs.

3 **Now you've made those changes, you can go out and buy some probiotics,** which are healthy bacteria in a capsule. They will only help you once you're off the sugar and eating plenty of greens. Probiotics aim to replace the missing good bacteria. Some probiotic preparations work better than others (for more on how to choose good ones, see Chapter 6), but they all have two inherent problems which mean that although they are very useful, they are not a total gut cure.

Problem number one is that most of the bacteria which live naturally in our gut are anaerobic. That means they thrive in an environment without oxygen. Producers of probiotics can't easily put a bacterium in a capsule if it is anaerobic; it will come into contact with the air, and die. So even a combination of all the best probiotics on the market today will only contribute about 20 per cent of the gut bug diversity we need.

Problem number two is that most of the good bacteria in probiotic capsules will simply pass through our gut and come out the other end. They help on the way, but they don't usually take root and implant themselves in the colon lining as we would like them to. If you're a gardener, think annuals not perennials; you need to keep re-planting every year. So most people who find that probiotics help them also find that the benefits fade when they stop taking them. But for many people, the benefits in terms of bowel function and general mental and physical well-being are significant enough that they do find it worthwhile to keep taking them long term. In hunter-gatherer times we would have got many of those good bugs from a huge variety of plants with some of the soil still on them.

I find there is one group of patients in whom probiotics **do** seem to "take root", and who derive lasting benefits from taking them just for a few weeks as a one-off. These are the people who were breastfed long term as babies. It makes a difference even well into old age. If someone was breastfed for a year or more (and 3 to 4 years is normal in many non-Western cultures), then the damage to their gut (due to antibiotics, the pill, stress, bad diet or infection) can usually be repaired in a matter of months. If people were not breastfed at all, gut recovery can take a couple of years, and is not always complete. (More on the magical properties of breastmilk in Chapter 5.)

The best probiotic to take is one that you keep changing. We still know so little about the microbiome that we can't yet reliably say, "This is the probiotic just right for YOU for all time." So keep trying different types (See the guidelines in Chapter 6) and keep changing to different combinations even if the first one you try works brilliantly. As with food, the key here is variety.

> **A word about "pre-biotics"**
>
> You may see this on the label, and they are usually a special type of sugar also known as FOS, Fructo-Oligo-Saccharides, that are supposed to feed the good bacteria with which they're combined in the capsule. I am not convinced they are always helpful; they make some people's abdominal wind and bloating worse. I suspect these "pre-biotics" feed the unfriendly bugs just as much as the friendly ones – so you might want to find a brand without any added FOS. Suck it and see.

If you've been on the probiotics for a couple of months, and you're sticking with lots of veg and zero sugar, it's time to add in a remedy or two to attack the unfriendly bugs. The ones that work most effectively for most people are caprylic acid (from coconut), grapefruit seed extract, and numerous herbal extracts including oregano oil, berberine, goldenseal root and plain old raw garlic. One at a time, rotate them. Here's why you mustn't rush, and why you must improve your diet and start the probiotics **before** you go for something like grapefruit seed extract or caprylic acid or any herb that targets the unfriendly bugs.

The "unfriendly bugs", who almost certainly include yeasts (single-celled fungi) as well as bacteria, have been making you feel lousy and "foggy headed" by virtue of the metabolic waste products they release into your system. If you kill them all at once, bang bang, without first starving them of sugar and preparing the ground with the friendly bugs (probiotics), they will release huge amounts of those same metabolic waste products as they die off. This is called "die-off" or the "Herxheimer reaction", and it can make you feel dreadful for several days. So don't do that to yourself; take the steps in the right order, and take your time.

If you have done all of the above over a 3–4 month period you will probably feel a whole lot better. If you don't, it may well be that you have a hidden food allergy; something you're eating is making you ill. The most common culprits are wheat, or possibly all the gluten grains (wheat, spelt, rye, barley and most oats), dairy products, sweetcorn (maize) and soya. You can try the experiment of leaving all these foods out and systematically reintroducing them into your diet, one food per day, noting down the effects. This is a scaled-down version of the "elimination diet" protocol, described in more detail in Becky's story in the Autumn chapter. Whichever foods you suspect, this process will only work reliably for you if you've followed the steps above – no sugar, more veg, some probiotics and some anti-bad-bugs remedies – first.

Spring Case History: Jonathan's Hay fever

Jonathan was in his early 40s when he came to see me. I heard him before I saw him, sneezing his head off in the waiting room at the far end of the corridor. He came into the consulting room scattering paper tissues from his sleeves. It was mid-May in central London. His eyes were red and streaming, and he was deeply fed up; it was getting worse, he told me, year-on-year.

Jonathan already knew that pollen was not the only culprit. He lived and worked in the city, but his parents had recently moved to the countryside, and he spent most weekends there. It was remarkable, he told me, how little he sneezed at their house.

"It's ridiculous," he said, "I'm surrounded by grass there, and trees and plants of all sorts; there must be masses of pollen. But although I do sneeze a bit there, it's much less than here in town. I come back to London on a Sunday evening and by Monday morning I'm like this again." He pointed to his red nose and sore, puffy eyes.

Hay fever, despite its name, was rare or unknown before the Industrial Revolution. The first description of it in the UK medical literature was in 1819, in a paper presented by Dr John Bostock (1772–1846) to the Medical and Chirugical (surgical) Society.[60] In Japan, where the Industrial Revolution occurred about 100 years later than in Britain, hay fever also appeared about 100 years later than in Britain.[61] But in Japan people developed allergic reactions to the pollen of Japanese trees, in particular the cedar tree. In the UK, similarly, people become allergic to the pollen of their local grasses or trees, though different people get ill at different parts of the hay fever season, depending on when their particular "demon pollen" is most plentiful in the air.

What's happening here is that particles of air pollution, primarily from vehicle exhaust fumes, are somehow causing people to have violent allergic reactions to an essentially harmless biological material that has been part of our natural environment for ever: plant pollen. This is an example of the phenomenon that Dr Claudia Miller of the University of Texas has called "TILT" – Toxicant-Induced Loss of Tolerance.[62] In other words, inherently toxic substances (in this case car fumes) are causing the body to react to an inherently harmless substance (in this case pollen) as though it were dangerous. This phenomenon is a big contributor to the rise of allergies in general, not just hay fever.

There are at least three possible mechanisms that have been suggested to explain why hay fever is worse in polluted urban areas:

Firstly, exhaust fumes damage the shell of pollen grains, so they split open and release their contents, namely pollen powder composed of particles so tiny that, unlike the whole pollen grain, they can enter our lungs. Secondly, many pollen grains can get stuck to a single particle of air pollution, thus making pollen more concentrated in urban air.[63] Thirdly, pollen grains released in a natural environment would simply fall to the earth and be absorbed into the ground or washed away by rain. But when they fall onto a concrete surface they can get blown around by the wind; they hang around longer, and don't disappear.

All these mechanisms suggest that air pollution is intensifying what would otherwise be a mild and transient immune response, and turning it into a disabling condition.

Jonathan didn't remember ever having had hay fever as a child or young adult, but he had two close relatives with asthma, and one with eczema, so he probably shared their "atopic" tendency. Atopy means the familial tendency to an over-reactive immune system in the upper respiratory tract and the skin, leading to allergic rhinitis (of which hay fever is one seasonal example), asthma and allergic dermatitis (eczema).

"It's not just the sneezing and the eyes now," he said. "I also feel sort of drugged with it, like I can't think clearly, and I can't function properly at work. And that's not just the antihistamines – I feel a bit like that even when I don't take them. The reason I'm here really is that I don't want to be taking antihistamines for three months of every year; I've been reading up about their long-term side effects."

Jonathan showed me a study he had printed off showing a link between dementia and long-term use of antihistamines.[64] He was quite right to be apprehensive.

"And anyway," he added, "if I take a high enough dose to actually stop the hay fever, it knocks me out completely, even the so-called non-drowsy ones. I just don't like the thought of what those drugs are doing to my brain – there has to be another way."

I took a detailed medical history from Jonathan, and discovered, as is often the way, that although it was the hay fever that was bothering him most, that certainly wasn't his only problem. He also had acne on his back, and he also had IBS. A stool test showed an almost complete absence of lactobacillus species (important friendly bacteria) and an overgrowth of two types of yeast. He was opening his bowels 4–5 times a day, with some urgency, and with soft, not properly formed stools.

"I thought that was normal," he said. "I've been like that for as long as I can remember. That's just me."

Jonathan was not thrilled to hear that the lungs, the skin and the immune system are profoundly affected by the state of the gut, and that the gut was where we had to start with treating his hayfever. (Ideally, of course, he would also have moved out of town to a less polluted area, but that wasn't practical for the foreseeable future.)

Jonathan agreed (only because he was desperate) to cut out his sugary snacks, including breakfast cereals, and to eat proper meals with fish, eggs, vegetables and whole grains rather than the white bread, white pasta and white rice he was living on. (Whole grains make some people's IBS better and others' worse – you have to Suck it and See – but a basic guideline is that if your gut is behaving badly, then the way you are eating now isn't working for you.)

I asked Jonathan to make these changes **slowly** to allow his gut and its TTCs to get used to new foods and more fibre, and to the withdrawal of sugar. He was, however, rather impatient, and made all the changes immediately. Unsurprisingly, he got diarrhoea, but within three or four days that had settled down, and, as he told me at our second session, "I'm only going two or three times a day, and it's proper formed poo!" He had brought a copy of the Bristol Stool Chart (terribly useful but not to be studied at meal-times) and pointed enthusiastically to a picture of the correctly shaped item.

"But I've lost a bit of weight," he said. He was thin, and could not afford to lose any weight. What he hadn't heard was my instruction to replace the calories from sugar with calories from healthy fats, such as avocados, nuts, seeds, hempseed oil (raw) and coconut oil (to fry with). Patients often don't register this, even though it's very important; perhaps surprisingly, many people find it easier to cut out bad foods than to put in new and better foods. It is vital to do both. With some good-quality pro-biotics and some grapefruit seed extract, Jonathan's gut continued to improve, till he hardly recognised himself. At our fourth session (by which time the hay fever season was well over, so we couldn't yet judge what impact we'd had on that) he declared himself free of IBS.

His acne, at that point, was just beginning to improve. It did clear, but it took several more months. You cannot clear the skin (of acne or eczema) without first treating the gut, but you need to know that the improvement in the skin will lag behind the improvement in the gut. That's how it works, from the inside out. Tough for teenagers, but Jonathan wasn't a teenager.

Our penultimate consultation was in April the following year. Jonathan's hay fever was milder but still present. He was trying to make plans to leave London; I could help him control what went into his mouth, and that helped, but I could do nothing about the air he inhaled. I had him on only two supplements now: Vitamin D because it calms down the over-reactive immune system, and Vitamin C because in high doses it reduced the severity of his hay fever symptoms.

At our final appointment, Jonathan told me that he had found a remedy for his hay fever which, on top of all the changes we had already made, more or less finished off the seasonal sneezes. It was: local, raw honey. Even though he was still in the city, he had found a beekeeper on an allotment nearby, who swore that he used honey from his hive to ward off his own hay fever. It made sense to Jonathan, and it worked for him too, and I have his permission to share it with other patients and with you. It is a natural form of desensitisation. But it must be LOCAL honey; the bees must live within half a mile of you, so they are feeding from the same local plants whose pollen is affecting you. Supermarket honey won't do. It is usually labelled "produce of more than one country".

"But isn't honey full of the dreaded SUGAR?" I hear you cry. Yes. But: (a) we had already successfully treated Jonathan's gut, so it was no longer crawling with hostile, sugar-grabbing yeasts, and (b) he was only taking half a teaspoon a day, and that now constituted his sole sugar intake, and (c) it was only for three or four months of the year and (d) life is the art of sensible compromise.

My thanks to Jonathan and the wise urban beekeeper. Let's preserve our bees; we need them for so many reasons.

Take-Home Tips For Spring

- Get up in time to have breakfast – you'll have a better day.

- Spring weather is notoriously unpredictable – eat according to the actual temperature, not the calendar!

- Grow salad leaves and sprouted seedlings on your windowsill.

- Spring clean your gut not your home.

- Exercise – this is the ideal time of year to start increasing your exercise level. But if you're finding that you just don't have the energy, ask your GP to check your thyroid hormone level.

- Weight loss – if you need to, again, this is the time to start. But do it slowly; if you lose weight quickly, you'll likely regain it quickly. Again, if you are struggling, ask your GP to test your thyroid. Be suspicious of a "borderline" result; ask them to test T4 as well as TSH.

- Watch out for people spraying pesticides and herbicides in your vicinity. Avoid them at all costs.

✍ Put neem powder on your cat or dog to prevent fleas – this is a safe alternative to toxic flea collars and insecticide drops, and is detailed in the Summer chapter on pages 110–111.

✍ In early spring, you might need to continue taking the "first-aid package" of winter supplements, to prevent coughs and colds, until mid-April.

CHAPTER 3

SUMMER

(June, July, August)

Make the most of it! This is the raw food season, so eat lots of salads. Here's a recipe for a simple salad dressing that will keep for a week in the fridge in a stoppered glass bottle. Squeeze a lemon and/or a lime, add some cold-pressed hempseed oil and/or olive oil, lots of crushed raw garlic and as much honey as you need to balance the sharpness of the lemon or lime. Gradually reduce the amount of honey you use, to train your taste buds away from sweet.

If you want to try being vegan for a while, this is the season to do it. There's such a huge variety of veg, that if you add in some whole grains such as rice, quinoa and buckwheat, and some peas, beans and nuts, and keep sprouting the seedlings on your windowsill (see pages 76–78), you should be fine at least till September. If you're a lean and hungry vegan, an avocado will fill the gap nicely.

What's In Season And Good To Eat?

A lot. Red and yellow peppers, cucumber, tomatoes, lettuce, other salad leaves, basil and many other herbs, celery, beetroot, radishes, new potatoes, courgettes, aubergines, broccoli, cauliflower, peas, mangetout, broad beans, French beans, runner beans, fennel, spinach, pak choi, chard, plums, peaches, cherries and berries. In August (it used to be September), pick your own blackberries. Wild salmon.

What's Out Of Season?

Oranges. Not much else!

Nutrients You Might Be Lacking

There's no reason to be deficient in any nutrients in summer, so long as you are eating plenty of raw food, and have supplemented as needed through winter and early spring. So you shouldn't have to take supplements in the summer unless you've got a particular health issue. But here's a caveat: **Vitamin D**. If the sun is shining, that's great, but it can only make Vitamin D in your skin if you expose plenty of skin to it, for plenty of time! That's our natural source of Vitamin D; the action of sunshine on our naked skin.

Sunlight acts on the cholesterol in our skin. The UVB (Ultraviolet B) rays convert the cholesterol into Vitamin D. So sunshine raises our level of Vitamin D while simultaneously using up some of our cholesterol. But to make useful amount of Vitamin D, we need to expose a large area of skin to the sun; more than just our hands and face. We need to be wearing shorts and short sleeves, so at least our arms and legs are exposed to the sun. Ideally most of the torso for some of the summer as well. The darker your skin, the more melanin it contains, and therefore the more sun exposure you need to make enough Vitamin D.

But what about skin cancer? That's discussed under the first hazard below.

Health Hazards Of Summer And How To Prevent Them

Sunburn

The relationship between sun exposure and skin cancer is not clear or simple. First of all, even though sunlight remains absolutely essential to our health and happiness, the sun may be more dangerous to our skin than it was 100 years ago. This is because of the depletion of the ozone layer around our planet, which in turn is due to our massive past production of synthetic chemicals such as CFCs (chlorofluorocarbons) and other aerosols. The ozone layer filters out the potentially damaging wavelengths of UVB sunlight. So sunlight does now pose more of a risk than it did, particularly in areas where the ozone layer is thinnest. This means we have to be more careful about **how** we expose our skin to the sun.

The main way to stay safe is to build up your sun exposure **very gradually**. It is common sense: don't turn up on a beach in southern Europe in August after spending the year covered up in Britain, and lie out in the sun all day in your bikini or swimming trunks. You will BURN. It is sunburn rather than suntan that increases the risk of skin cancer. Sunburn is a form of radiation damage and radiation is carcinogenic. It can also make you quite ill in the short term; sunstroke is a very unpleasant acute illness that is potentially dangerous in its own right.

To avoid burning, you need to build up a tan slowly. In response to a little sunshine, the melanocytes in the skin will start to produce the brown pigment melanin, which is actually protective against sunburn. So roll your sleeves up and wear shorts as soon it's bearable to do so in the UK – April or May. Get outside at every opportunity. Even a few minutes a day will help. This mirrors the way we would have tanned by working in the fields before the industrial revolution. Then increase your exposure time. When the sun is strong, the parts of your body that haven't been exposed for a long time need five minutes maximum on the first day, then 10 on the next, 15 on the next and so on. When you cover up, do so with loose, white, cotton clothing.

The process of tanning is not chemically the same as the process of making Vitamin D, but both processes require direct exposure. Tanning builds up the level of protective melanin in your skin. But be aware that if you are a fair-skinned, freckled redhead then you probably cannot tan, and are likely to just burn; you have to cover up, and will need to get your Vitamin D from eating lots of oily fish and/or from supplements.

Sunscreens

What about sunscreens? Surely they are the most effective protection against sunburn?

There are two problems with sunscreen creams. The first is, if they are strong enough to stop you burning (e.g. factor 45), they are also blocking the sun from converting cholesterol into Vitamin D in your skin. The second is more serious: most sunscreens contain toxic ingredients such as titanium dioxide, oxybenzone and octyl methoxycinnamate, which are absorbed through your skin into your body.[65,66] Some people even suspect that the increase in skin cancers is actually due to the rising use of sunscreens rather than to the sun itself.[67]

I suspect it is a bit of both. There are a few sunscreens which are relatively non-toxic, such as those made (at time of writing) by Green People. You can build up your sun exposure gradually using these safer sunscreens initially (check the ingredients list with a magnifying glass), and eventually letting go of them. And if you are going to travel to hot countries in southern Europe, you might consider doing so in spring or autumn, rather than at the height of summer. You will get plenty of sun, but with less risk of burning.

There are three main types of skin cancer. They are: basal cell carcinoma (BCC or rodent ulcer), squamous cell carcinoma (SCC) and malignant melanoma. The first two, although technically cancers, are effectively "benign" in that they do not spread (metastasise) to distant parts of the body.[68] They tend to remain "in situ", i.e. in the place where they begin, and they grow very slowly. They are usually removed at an early stage for cosmetic reasons, and only become a serious problem if they are completely neglected and allowed to grow unchecked, which is very rare these days.

The third type, malignant melanoma, is the one people are really worried about. It is an aggressive, rapidly growing cancer of the melanocytes, the cells in our skin that make the brown pigment melanin. Melanomas can metastasise to other parts of the body, including the liver, and can be potentially life-threatening if they are not caught early. Catching them early means noticing any changes in moles in your skin. If one appears or enlarges suddenly, or starts bleeding, go and show it to your GP immediately. This is something that the NHS is very good at; you will see a dermatologist within two weeks, and if it is remotely suspicious it will be removed, and a pathologist will study it under the microscope to determine whether it is a melanoma or not. The vast majority of lumps and bumps on the skin, even dark and itchy ones, do not turn out to be melanomas.

There are several studies about the incidence of melanomas and their relationship to sun exposure, and the results are not always what you would expect, or what the manufacturers of sunscreens would have you believe. At least one eminent professor of dermatology thinks we are worrying far too much about the sun.[69] And a study from the National Cancer Institute showed that avoiding the sun actually increased the risk of death from melanoma; those who got more sun exposure lived significantly longer.[70]

Insect bites

Whether it's Scottish midges or tropical mosquitoes, here are five things you can do to discourage them from biting you:

1 Take a high-dose Vitamin B complex, containing 100 mg of each of the major B vitamins. Insects don't like the taste at all. But remember, the vitamin B2 (riboflavin) in the B complex will turn your urine bright yellow. This doesn't matter at all. But don't pee in the pool – you'll be spotted instantly! Add to this a very high dose (500 mg twice daily) of vitamin B1 (thiamine) even though there is some thiamine in your B complex. Insects **really** dislike thiamine.*

2 Insects also dislike garlic, so eating plenty of raw garlic will keep them away.

3 Stay right off sugar. Insects love to bite you when you taste sweet, so if you avoid sugar, they are more likely to avoid you; they'll go and bite the person who's just had an ice cream.

4 Cover up if you're outside at dawn or dusk, using white or pale-coloured clothing. Don't wear bright yellow; insects will think you're a flower, and come to visit.

5 Avoid stagnant water like ponds and puddles; mozzies congregate there.

---

* I am grateful to Dr Charles Forsyth for the information about this use of vitamin B1.

My patients come back from holidays reporting either no bites or very few bites on this regime. If you do get bitten, safe alternatives to antihistamines are quercetin, boswellia (frankincense) and curcumin (turmeric), available in capsules from your local health-food shop. They are all natural, herbal anti-inflammatories.

> ### Natural homemade insect repellent
>
> Conventional insect repellents are full of nasty chemicals, but you can make a safe, totally natural insect repellent at home. There are five essential oils that help: geranium, lavender, ylang-ylang, pettigrain and neroli. Mix them into a spray bottle with water, or into some coconut oil with 2% neem oil, also a natural insect repellent. Neem doesn't smell too good, but the essential oils (which smell great!) should cover that up. (Contrary to popular belief, citronella doesn't help very much.)*

Tick bites are a particular problem. Some ticks (but by no means all) carry the microbe that causes Lyme disease. Ticks are found in wooded areas where there are sheep and deer. Get your travelling companion to check your body for ticks – they hang on, and you can't feel them. Remove them with a special tick-removing kit; you can buy these at a camping shop or online. Then return the favour! Use all the advice above for repelling insects, but don't bank on it where ticks are concerned; take the kit along as well as the garlic, B vitamins and essential oils.

---

* I am grateful to Dr Jayne Donegan for the information about these essential oils.

If you get stung by a **bee or wasp or hornet**, and you are prone to allergic reactions to such bites, obviously seek medical help urgently. These stings are particularly hazardous if they occur in the region of the mouth/lips/throat; if you start to swell up in that area, dial 999.

Nits/headlice

Kids catch lice at school, and it's **not** a reflection on their hygiene – in fact, lice attach more easily to clean hair than to greasy hair! Nits are the eggs laid by the lice.

Most of the stuff sold in chemists to kill headlice is toxic. Of course it is – it's insecticide. Insecticides are neurotoxins; they damage the nervous system most of all. The scalp has a very rich blood supply, with lots of blood vessels right near the surface. That's why the head bleeds so profusely when it's cut. This means that the innocent-looking, nicely scented, cleverly named gunk you are rubbing into your little one's scalp is being absorbed, through their skin, straight into their bloodstream. And it's bad for them.

Here's the alternative: Order a Bug Buster Kit very cheaply from CHC (Community Hygiene Concern), a charity who make the best nit combs and lice combs (not the same thing) and who will also send you full instructions on what to do, and information on the life cycle of the louse, which determines when you do it. Tel: 01908 261501 or 01908 561928. Shampoo and rinse, rub in lots of conditioner, and use CHC's combs in turn to physically remove all the nits and lice. No chemicals needed. And it actually works better than the toxic insecticides.[71] Combing the little blighters out like this only works in wet, conditioner-soaked hair. You can't catch 'em dry.

If you've done the job, but you just **know** that tomorrow at school your child is going to sit next to little Johnny who still has headlice, what can you do? You can let your child's hair dry with the conditioner still on. Don't rinse it off. Then it will be too slippery for all but the most determined of lice to attach to. If the hair is long, plait it tight; that also makes it harder for the lice to get a grip. (You can also tell kids not to put their heads together, but there's no point; they won't remember.)

Pet fleas

Dogs and cats get fleas. The standard treatment/prevention approach involves flea collars, or drops of liquid placed on the animal's fur. The drops are insecticide, and the flea collar is impregnated with insecticides. So both these methods expose you, your children and your pet to insecticides. Insecticides are very powerful chemicals – they have to be. Insects are tough, and any chemical that can kill them is harmful to all biological systems, and can damage the health of mammals – that's us. In particular, insecticides damage the nervous system, endocrine (hormone) system and reproductive system.

There are safe, non-toxic alternatives which are effective. I will tell you about them below. But first, what will the vet say? The vet will say: "It's only harmful for the first 48 hours. After that your toddler can stroke the animal." When you ask, as I have done many times, "Then how come the insecticide keeps killing fleas for three months? How can it be gone/harmless within two days, yet remain effective for three months?" you won't get an answer.

Some people have liver enzyme systems strong enough to

detoxify and remove these chemicals, up to a certain point. Many people don't. This is just genetic difference. I guess vets tend to be people with really strong detox enzyme systems; they couldn't get through veterinary training safely otherwise, as they handle so many chemicals. Hence perhaps their laissez-faire attitude. But to be fair, they weren't taught about the health hazards of insecticides at veterinary school, just as I wasn't at medical school.

Safe, non-toxic flea treatment and prevention

A safe and effective alternative is neem powder, the powdered bark of the neem tree. It is an ancient and modern Indian herbal remedy, and it works. Get it from any reputable supplier of herbal remedies. Rub it into your cat or dog, all over. Three things will happen:

1) You will have a green pet for a day or so. Don't worry, that's ok.
2) The fleas will die.
3) The cat/dog will lick the neem powder off, and therefore it will also kill any parasitic worms in the animal's gut, i.e. it acts as a worming powder.

You can use neem preventatively too; don't wait for a flea infestation!

There is another method too, and this one you **can** get from the vet. It is a white liquid called "Program" (American spelling) which you mix with your pet's food once a month. It is a preventive not a cure, and it's not an insecticide. It doesn't kill the fleas, but it sterilises them, so any flea that bites your pet becomes unable to breed. So it drops off harmlessly, and you never get a flea infestation.

You can use either or both of these methods, and it makes sense to start in March before the weather begins to get warmer; fleas like it hot.

Burning food on the bbq

It's fine to barbecue food, but please don't burn it. Burning meat produces carcinogenic substances such as acrylamide and nitrosamines.[72,73]

Pesticide spraying

As in the Spring chapter, pages 78–80: avoid it.

Using plastic water bottles

Phthalates, BPA (BisPhenol A) and other plasticiser chemicals are released from plastic water bottles if you are carrying them around on a hot summer's day. They get into the water. You don't want to be drinking these plasticisers; they are Endocrine Disrupting Compounds (they mess with your hormones) and are potentially carcinogenic too. Plastic water bottles exposed to the sun through car windows are particularly bad news. Plastic is not only clogging up the oceans, it's poisoning us directly too. Use glass bottles, protected by a padded container which you can get from any camping shop. Unfortunately, schools and some other public institutions don't allow glass bottles. So an alternative is metal flasks, but only for water. Don't put juice in them; the acid can leach the nickel out of stainless steel (see page 271).

Salt loss

It's easy to forget that we lose salt as well as water by sweating in hot weather. Do replace the salt as well as the water.

Tropical travel

Malaria and other insect-borne diseases, travellers' diarrhoea and jet lag are among the potential hazards of tropical travel. Artemisia is a traditional herbal treatment for **malaria**, now modified to the drug Artemisinin for the same purpose. It **may** have value as a preventer as well,[74] if used in addition to the methods described above for preventing mosquitoes from biting. But some malaria parasites are already developing resistance to it and to other anti-malarials. None of these methods is foolproof, and malaria is a very serious disease. So if, like many people, you are reluctant to use conventional malaria-preventing drugs, I would simply recommend not travelling to malarial areas during their malarial season.

There are plenty of other tropical diseases transmitted by biting insects, and while the methods described on page 107 will reduce your chances of being bitten, they are not a guarantee. Mosquito nets can be helpful, but most of them come impregnated with insecticides which, as we have seen, are toxic.

To reduce your chances of getting tropical **diarrhoea**, observe the following six points:

1 Eat only well-cooked, piping-hot food; avoid salads.

2 Fruit – only if you peel it yourself, and/or wash it in safe, clean water.

3 Avoid eating ice.

4 Regarding bottled water, check the top. Only trust it if it's sealed.

5 Iodine drops or iodine crystals can be used as a water-purifier.

6 Take a probiotic every day, and double the dose if you do get a tummy bug.

Jet lag

If you are flying a long way east or west, some degree of jet lag is unavoidable. But there are a few things that help to reduce it:

1 Drink lots of water on the flight, and don't eat too much airline food.

2 Take lots of Vitamin C on the flight; 500 mg every two hours is good, **if** you have checked before you fly that your bowel can tolerate that much. Most people can.

3 Eat a good meal as soon as you can after landing, to help "ground" you in your new time zone.

As you will see from Graham's case history in Chapter 7, jet lag is by no means the most hazardous aspect of flying. You might, when you've read it, want to rediscover the delights of holidaying in England, Ireland, Scotland or Wales. What's bad for the planet tends to be bad for the person directly too. But first, let's meet Jeanette.

Summer Case History: Jeanette's Hot Flushes

Jeanette was 54 when she came to see me. She was a Nursing Sister at a large hospital, and was three years past the menopause (more about menopause in Chapter 5). She was experiencing about 10–12 hot flushes every day, and said they were bearable in winter but completely intolerable in summer. "At least in the winter I can rush outdoors and cool off," she said. Her GP had offered HRT (hormone replacement therapy) but Jeanette had refused, because of her family history. Her mother, maternal aunt, sister and a cousin had all had breast cancer, and in three of those four relatives the cancer had been the hormone-sensitive type, i.e. stimulated by an excess of the female hormone oestrogen. When Jeanette explained this to the GP, she understood and agreed with her decision, but had nothing else to offer.

Giving Jeanette Vitamin E helped considerably, as it helps with most problems associated with the menstrual cycle or menopause; by the time Jeanette's blood level of Vitamin E had normalised, which took nearly 6 months, the flushes had reduced to about four or five per day, and were milder. It was important for Jeanette to take the right kind of Vitamin E. Naturally occurring Vitamin

E is in fact eight substances, not one, and all eight sub-types occur together in food, and work together; we need them all. Yet most Vitamin E supplements sold in the UK contain only one type of Vitamin E: alpha tocopherol. Why? Because alpha tocopherol is easy to synthesise. But why synthesise it anyway? Why make it in a lab when you can extract the whole eight-part vitamin from plants? The answer is £. It's cheaper to make alpha tocopherol. I suggested that Jeanette take "Gamma Vitamin E"; at time of writing, the one made by *Life Extension* contains all eight sub-types of Vitamin E.

Jeanette's diet was not bad considering she worked shifts; she made herself packed lunches with fresh fruit and veg, and avoided eating in the hospital canteen. The only change I made was to ask her to increase her intake of foods rich in Vitamin E: eggs, avocados, nuts, seeds and lettuce. Her initial Vitamin E level was so low that food alone would not have normalised it, hence the need for the supplement, but food would remain important for maintenance once she stopped the supplement.

I also made sure that Jeanette had plenty of zinc, magnesium, iodine, Vitamin C, Vitamin D and all the B vitamins. They all help with the symptoms of menopause in their own right, and Vitamin C supports the action of Vitamin E too. I suggested that Jeanette wore only natural cotton clothing, as it is cooler and more breathable than synthetic fabrics. And she agreed to cut down her cups of tea from an astonishing ten daily to four daily, and this helped too.

Jeanette only told me at our third consultation that she had been taking fish oil supplements (omega 3) for many years, over the counter. She had heard they were good for the brain and for breast cancer prevention. This is true, up to a point. But the body needs good omega 6 oils as well as omega 3, and many people are unwittingly overdosing on the omega 3s and thus getting out of balance. When I measured Jeanette's blood levels of essential fatty acids (EFAs) I found her levels of the omega 3s (EPA and DHA) were over the top, but she was very low on the healthy omega 6 EFAs (GLA and DGLA). So I gave her some Evening Primrose Oil, a good source of the right type of omega 6, and within a few weeks she noted a further reduction in the hot flushes. On my advice she stopped the fish oil supplement, but made sure to eat oily fish at least twice a week.

Another recommendation that Jeanette found helpful was a contemporary meditation practice called MBSR, Mindfulness-Based Stress Reduction. The hypothalamus in the brain does a bit of a meltdown at the menopause, and the slightest stressful thought or event, however minor, can spark off a hot flush. MBSR seems to reduce that hair-trigger sensitivity in the brain. Jeanette did the full eight-week course of MBSR in a group with a real teacher, which is infinitely better than any online version. It didn't reduce the frequency of the hot flushes, which were already much less frequent than when she first came, but she reported that it made them far less distressing, and greatly increased her overall sense of well-being.

At our fourth appointment Jeanette described the hot flushes as "30 per cent of what they were; not gone, but much more live-able with". Jeanette declared herself happy, but there was one more task to be done: breast cancer prevention. For this it is important always to maintain a good level of iodine, selenium, Vitamin C[75,76] and Vitamin D, as well as a good balance of the omega 3 and omega 6 EFAs. It is also a good idea to avoid tight or underwired bras, which impede the free flow of lymph from the breast to the lymph nodes in the armpits.[77] Lymph is a body fluid similar to blood, but without the red blood cells, that flows in a system of vessels like veins from all our tissues back to the heart. It passes through lymph nodes, collections of white blood cells which are a vital part of the immune system, trapping cancer cells and dodgy microbes.

For breast cancer prevention it is also vital to avoid the toxins which are implicated in breast cancer, such as pesticides, insecticides, herbicides, plasticisers like BPA and the heavy metals mercury, aluminium and nickel. (See Chapter 7 for more on this.) Finally, there are certain foods that are thought to be protective, such as grapefruit, raspberries and the brassica vegetables[78] (broccoli, cauliflower, cabbage, kale, Brussels sprouts and watercress). Jeanette now eats some of these every day.

Jeanette comes for a nutritional check-up once a year, and remains very well ten years on. At a recent annual check-up she brought along her partner, Kath, who is the same age but had sailed through the menopause with no hot flushes at all. Kath, however, suffered from recurrent cold sores, and most of the session was devoted to cold sore treatment and prevention. Here is a summary of the most important nutrients for fighting off cold sores; bear in mind, though, that as with most health problems, prevention works better than cure.

Cold sores

Cold sores are caused by the herpes simplex virus. Once you've had it, it lives in the nerve endings, and remains mostly dormant, but will flare up and cause visible cold sores if you become tired or stressed, both of which states weaken the immune system and thereby make you "run down". Harsh direct sunlight can trigger an eruption too. There are three nutrients which together are excellent at preventing cold sores. They are:

Vitamin B12, taken as a supplement in its own right – there's not enough in a B complex to do the trick. **Lysine**, an amino acid that's found in most protein foods, but not in sufficient amounts for this purpose, so use a Lysine supplement. And lastly, **Vitamin E** again, both as a supplement to take, as above, and also in liquid form, applied directly to the cold sore area, several times a day. Applied at the first tingle, it lowers the chance of the cold sore erupting. Applied to an already-present cold sore, it speeds the healing and reduces scarring. Kath carries a bottle around with her now. It's oily and smelly but it works. At time of writing, Solgar make a liquid Vitamin E which is fine for this purpose.

Take-Home Tips For Summer

In very hot weather, if you are sweating a lot, do remember to replace the salt as well as the water. Drink water from glass, not plastic. It's better to drink water between meals rather than with meals. Drinking water with a meal dilutes your digestive enzymes. If you feel thirsty after a meal, chances are that what you ate was too sweet, too salty or too dry. Or you hadn't had any water to drink for too long **before** the meal. Keep healthily hydrated; the only cold drink you need is water. Filter your tap water to remove chlorine and other nasties – see Chapter 7 for advice on water filters.

- It's ok to have a siesta – an afternoon nap. Most people in most places have done this from time immemorial.

- If you must dry-clean your clothes or curtains (and I'd much rather you didn't, because dry-cleaning chemicals are so toxic that some countries won't even allow a dry-cleaner's shop next to a food shop), then please do it in summer, so you can hang the dry-cleaned clothes outside for at least 48 hours before you bring them into your house. This enables some of the dry-cleaning fluids to "out-gas" from your clothes.

- If your child has nits/lice or your pet has fleas, check out the tips for how to deal with that naturally and safely (pages 109–112).

- If you are planning to fly off somewhere hot, check out the Tropical Travel tips on pages 113–114. And for flying anywhere, take Vitamin C at frequent intervals on the flight, and put a mask from "Angel Fleet" in your hand luggage, just in case (www.angelfleet.net).

◢ Even if you are holidaying in the UK, biting insects can still be a problem; see the natural insect-repellent techniques on pages 107–108.

◢ Get some sun on your skin – but safely. Details on pages 103–105. If your Vitamin D level is so low that you are needing to take Vitamin D supplements even in summer, take them in the evening. Then you'll still be able to make the most of the summer sunshine. If you take Vitamin D in the mornings, it raises your blood level of Vitamin D, so your body thinks you've got plenty, and your skin won't bother making it from the sunshine, which is the better source. Vitamin D is also better absorbed in the evening. But hopefully by next year your levels will have normalised, and you won't need the supplements through the summer.

CHAPTER 4

AUTUMN

(September, October, November)

Much of the bounty of summer is still around in early autumn, in terms of fruit and veg, sunshine and energy. Harvest it; it won't last! Be conscious of maintaining the health of your immune system in September and October, so you don't get ill in November/December. By November/December you may need the immune system support package described on pages 67–68 – don't wait for the winter bugs; get your retaliation in early!

What's In Season And Good To Eat?

Still quite a lot:

- **Pumpkins and all sorts of squashes.** Full of carotene (you don't need to get the huge ones; smaller is better).

- **Parsnips, carrots, kale, celery, leeks, spinach, chard, runner beans**

- **Brussels sprouts and winter cabbage in late Autumn.** Still some good broccoli, cauliflower, beetroot, cucumber and tomatoes.

- **Apples and pears.** You can cook them if you have a delicate digestive system.

- **Figs, grapes, autumn raspberries and late plums.** Don't overdose on figs and grapes; they're very high in sugar, as are dates.

- **Wild blackberries.** In September there may still be some to pick. They grow in most woods, fields and parks in the UK, and they're free. You don't need to get the sprayed, squishy, plastic-packed ones from the supermarket.

About fruit

Apples and pears ripen in early autumn in the UK. Sadly, the huge variety of types of apple that we used to grow has been greatly reduced by the industrialisation of agriculture over the past few decades.[79] Nevertheless, it still possible and important to get UK-grown apples and pears in season. You have to look carefully when you are shopping, though; some supermarkets will stock apples and pears from the other side of the world even in the midst of the British apple season. Don't buy them – their transport here is polluting the planet and contributing to climate change. It's totally unnecessary (but highly profitable).

How much fruit should you eat? What does "in moderation" mean? Well, if you restrict yourself to eating fruit only when it's in season, and to having only fresh, whole fruit rather than fruit juice or dried fruit, you should be fine. Fresh, whole fruit contains water, fibre, many excellent phytonutrients including Vitamin C and, yes, some sugar. The problem with sugar overdose arises primarily with fruit juice and dried fruit, as you will see below.

When you make fruit juice out of fruit, you remove all the fibre. Fibre not only provides bulk or "roughage" and food for the friendly TTCs in your gut (see Chapter 2), it also slows down the rate at which the sugar is absorbed from the gut into the bloodstream. By preventing the "sugar rush" which takes such a heavy toll on the pancreas and liver, it reduces your risk of developing type 2 diabetes. However, if you drink a glass of apple juice there is no fibre left in it to do that job. Furthermore, an average glass of apple juice contains the juice of about NINE apples – so it contains nine times more sugar than you'd get from just eating an apple. You couldn't eat nine apples in a day, still less in the two minutes it takes to swallow a glass of apple juice. You'd get terrible gut ache. It's AN apple a day that keeps the doctor away, not nine!

Fruit juice is bad news: it's a guaranteed sugar overdose.[80] And commercially produced fruit juice is not going to retain all the nutrients of the fresh fruit; it is often made from concentrate. It's been processed, stored, transported, and contains juices from several different countries, so it's very hard to trace its origins. If you compare the taste of commercial orange juice with the taste of an actual orange – well, it's not the same. And what about the cartons that fruit juice comes in? What are they lined with? Is it safe?

Dried fruit is equally problematic. Here, it is the water that has been removed, leaving the fibre, only a few nutrients and a lot of concentrated sugar. So raisins, sultanas, dried figs, dried apricots and so on – they're all too sweet to be eaten regularly or in large amounts. Furthermore, if they're not organic then they are coated in preservatives like sulphur dioxide. This is not good for you, and it's not necessary either; drying fruit is itself a method of preservation, and has been going on for thousands of years just fine without sulphur dioxide. As a method of food preservation it was useful back in the day when people ran out of food in the winter, but that's not the situation in the West now. And sulphur dioxide can trigger asthma attacks in some sensitive individuals.[81]

For most people, one or two pieces of fresh fruit a few days a week is fine. Regarding the government's "five a day" advice, I would say two things:

1 It should be about double that number, and

2 Only one or two of those portions should be fruit. Fruit and veg are not equal, and many of us are eating too much fruit and not enough veg.

Fruit has been bred to be much sweeter than it used to be, i.e. much sweeter than the fruit of the original wild tree/bush/vine.[82] Seedless grapes when they first appeared in the 1970s were so sour they would make you squirm – till you got used to them. However, they were safe and healthy and not contributing to the diabetes epidemic. But those grapes today – well, in terms of sugar content, they're almost like eating sweets. Fruit growers have done this because sugar is addictive. It sells; we keep coming back for more.

So, as I said in the Introduction, moderation with fruit means not having it all year round, just when it's in season. Berries are less sweet than most other fruit; you can cope with more, and they have many health benefits.

So far I've been generalising about fruit intake, but of course people vary. Some people have a condition called "fructose intolerance", or, more accurately, fructose malabsorption, and any amount of fruit upsets their stomach. But this is unusual. Other people think they have this problem but they don't, they simply can't eat fruit **together with other food**. To explain:

Most food spends 2–4 hours in your stomach before being shunted on down to the small intestine for the next phase of digestion. Fruit, however, if eaten on its own, sails through the system much faster, as it needs very little digestion. So it makes sense to eat fruit on its own, at least 20–30 minutes before a meal, rather than as a dessert. This is one of the useful insights of the Hay diet: the theory is that fruit eaten with/after a meal gets stuck in the stomach for hours, and putrefies, producing uncomfortable gassiness, and sometimes diarrhoea or constipation later on. Eaten on its own, they say, it doesn't do this.

The theory makes sense, but the only way to see if it applies to you is, as ever: Suck it and See. Try eating fruit only on an empty stomach (i.e. at least four hours after eating and at least 30 minutes before the next meal) for a few days and see if your gut becomes happier. The easiest way to do this is to have your fruit first thing in the morning, at least 30 minutes before your main breakfast. If you are dealing with gut dysbiosis (see page 83) you may need to cut fruit out completely **for a while**, as part of being strictly sugar-free. But not forever!

If you're still not sure, it is possible to do a breath test for fructose malabsorption. Your GP may agree to arrange this if your gut symptoms are severe, or otherwise, at time of writing, Biolab in central London will do this test if a practitioner refers you.

Having said all that, bear in mind that fruit is not the only (or remotely the worst) source of fructose. If you're still eating processed, packaged food, you will find "corn syrup" – very high in fructose – or indeed fructose itself listed on many an ingredients list. And it will be a much higher dose than you would get from eating a piece of fresh fruit. Fructose is sugar, sugar is an addictive drug: Just Say No.

What's Out Of Season?

Most foods are still good in early autumn. But by mid-November you should be cutting back on the salads and starting to have most of your food cooked, including most of the veg, as per the Winter chapter.

Nutrients You Might Be Lacking

Again, not many in September/October, but by late October your supply of Vitamin D from the summer sun may well be running out, unless you eat a lot of oily fish (and digest it well). This is a good time to get your friendly local GP to test your Vitamin D level – see page 53 for details of how to go about this.

Health Hazards Of Autumn And How To Prevent Them

Colds and flu

In late October/early November, colds and flu begin. Protect your-self and your kids with the "nutritional first-aid package" described on pages 67–68.

Moulds

The mould count goes up high in September, and this affects people in numerous ways, contributing to respiratory symptoms, joint pains and more. Moulds flourish inside most houses in the UK. This is because we have a damp climate, produce water vapour by cooking, bathing, showering and breathing, and then close our double-glazed windows to "keep the heat in". This leads to conden-sation, and moulds love these damp conditions. Once the mould has become visible as black patches in your bathroom/kitchen/ bedroom, it is already quite severe.

What is not widely known is that mould gives off chemical substances which are every bit as toxic as synthetic ones. People can actually become ill from spending too much time in a mouldy bathroom/bedroom/kitchen. The safest way to clean mould off is with old-fashioned Borax solution. However, it is best to prevent it building up in the first place. Below are a few tips to avoid growth of mould in your home.

Moulds do not thrive in hot dry conditions, for example near the Mediterranean/in southern Europe, so that is the climate you want to try and mimic in your home. This means, contrary to current thinking, that you need to have the windows open and, in the day-time in cold weather, the heating on. I'm afraid that's right – windows open and heating on. This will increase the air circulation and create hot, dry conditions where it is difficult for mould to grow. Visitors will say, "But the heat's going out the window!" and you say, "Yes, but so are the mould spores and mould toxins."

I appreciate that this is ecologically problematic, but it may be imperative for your health, particularly if your lungs or your joints are the issue. Many people with asthma get noticeably worse in the mould season, as we'll see in Becky's case history opposite. You can and should offset the slightly increased carbon footprint by planting trees, through The Woodland Trust, Trees For Life or other similar charities. In almost all situations, what's good for the planet is good for the person, but this is an unfortunate exception.

In your bathroom you need an extractor fan, and some form of heating in winter. You also ideally need an extractor hood above the cooker in the kitchen. In office buildings, old air conditioning systems, or those that are only infrequently cleaned and serviced, may also be a source of mould intoxication (this is one of many causes of "Sick Building Syndrome").

Note that **house dust mites (HDM)** feed on moulds, so measures to reduce mould will also help to reduce HDM. When you get out of bed in the morning, turn the duvet right back for at least an hour to let the night-time sweat evaporate. Otherwise moulds will have a field day in your bed, and the dust mites ditto. This is especially important for children with asthma and/or eczema, almost all of whom are allergic to the HDM. For further info on reduction of HDM, check out The Healthy House (see Resources section, page 333).

Autumn Case History: Becky's Asthma

Becky, aged 15, came to see me with her mother, Andrea. Becky had been diagnosed with asthma some three or four years previously, having become wheezy and breathless most nights and mornings. During the day at school she was not too bad, but needed her inhalers in order to play sport. Most of the family had hay fever but Becky did not.

Andrea told me that as a small child Becky had suffered severely with eczema. "She was covered in it. We had to tie mittens on her hands or she would scratch till she bled." Becky still had traces of the eczema visible in the elbow creases and behind her knees, but that was all.

Asthma, eczema and hay fever are together known as "atopy". Hay fever is really a special case of "allergic rhinitis"; the streaming nose may occur in autumn in those who react to mould, in spring in those with hay fever, or all year round in some people who haven't figured out what food or chemical or allergen they are reacting to. The "atopic tendency" usually runs in families, although all three conditions are becoming much commoner. When I was eight I was the only child in my school with asthma. Now every primary school classroom has a shelf for children's inhalers. The increase in the prevalence of asthma is due partly to outdoor air pollution, but in Becky's case this was probably not a major factor, since she lived in a small village.

I asked, as delicately as possible, whether there was a lot of dust at home. "Oh, loads," replied Andrea cheerfully. (Becky didn't speak much initially. She was in the "all adults are a waste of space" phase, although by age 17 she had become very friendly and chatty; these stages do pass.) "We live in a big old farmhouse, all wood and rugs and dark stone corners – there's dust everywhere!"

"What about in Becky's bedroom?" I asked.

"Same," Andrea said. "But it's toasty warm since we had the double glazing put in a few years ago."

I explained that some people, including most asthmatics, have an allergic reaction to house dust and/or the house dust mite (HDM), a tiny insect, invisible to the naked eye, that lives in dusty places but also in some quite clean places. And that the house dust mite feeds on moulds, and moulds love damp places. And that if the double-glazed windows were mostly closed – Andrea confirmed that they were – then dampness would build up in the house from people showering, bathing, cooking and simply breathing out.

Becky's asthma, said Andrea, was clearly at its worst in September. That's when the mould count is highest. HDMs are there all year round, but may be highest in September too because they feed on moulds (and human skin flakes. Yuck). The wheezing was a bit better by December/January, and much improved by April/May. From May to August Becky could manage without her inhalers, but as soon as autumn came she needed them again.

"So can I get rid of that manky old rug from my bedroom?" asked Becky, brightening up.

"Yes indeed," I said. "Rugs and carpets hold dust and dust mites."

Andrea looked horrified. The rug was apparently some kind of heirloom.

"Maybe it could go in another room?" I enquired. And that was agreed. Andrea and her husband worked full time, and she made it clear that she wasn't going to spend her time cleaning the old, rambling house.

"Fair enough," I said, "I think we don't really need to worry much about most of the house. It's just Becky's bedroom that matters. That's where she spends most of her time at home, right?"

"Yes, indeed."

I made it clear that no cleaning chemicals were required, simply regular damp-dusting of surfaces, vacuuming the floor and keeping the windows open 24 hours, with the heating on if necessary (explanation on pages 129–130). And that Becky should fold her duvet right back every morning and allow the bed to air for an hour before covering it up again. There's a slight dilemma here; duvet off all the time means dust settling on the sheets: bad. But duvet on all the time means that dampness (from night-time sweat) cannot evaporate, so moulds and house-dust mites thrive. Bad. So a good compromise is duvet off for the first hour of the day and then back on again.

I also recommended cotton bedding, and a HDM-proof cover on the mattress; I told Andrea she could order this from The Healthy House (see Resources section, page 333). And that the sheets needed washing once a week at 60° C, the minimum temperature required to kill the HDM. I hate making extra house-work for people, but such is life. It is mostly the minuscule faeces – droppings – of the HDM that trigger asthma and eczema in susceptible people, and that's what needs vacuuming up on a regular basis.

Finally, the pillows needed to be replaced every three months. I know that seems excessive, but they quickly fill up with HDM; after a few months, a significant percentage of the weight of a pillow is composed of house dust mite. It used to be thought that fewer HDMs accumulated in synthetic pillows, but a study in the

British Journal of Medicine proved just the opposite; feather pillows gathered fewer HDMs, weight-for-weight, than synthetic ones.[83] And of course feather pillows don't outgas the synthetic chemicals which may also exacerbate asthma.

Mattresses also gather HDMs, but you can't keep changing the mattress, so putting a HDM-proof cover on it is as good as it gets. Some parents of kids with asthma and eczema do vacuum the seams of their children' mattresses every week or even every day, but no one in Becky's family was ever going to do that, and I don't blame them; life's too short.

I asked Becky how she'd feel about damp-dusting her bedroom, and she rolled her eyes as only teenagers can. But in fact she did it, and most of the other changes I suggested, as above, were implemented too.

When I saw Becky for a second consultation she was about 30 per cent improved; a noticeable difference, but not yet sufficient to stop the inhalers. Test results showed that Becky had very low levels of magnesium in her cells. Magnesium is a natural muscle relaxant, and the bronchioles – the tiny tubes that carry air into and out of the lungs – are made of muscle. It is involuntary muscle, i.e. we cannot control it consciously in the way we can control our arm or leg muscles. It is the bronchioles that constrict – go into spasm – in an asthma attack. When Becky's bronchioles went into spasms, narrowing the space available for air to pass through, they could not relax again properly with such low levels of magnesium.

I asked Becky to raise her magnesium levels by taking a magnesium supplement, doing Epsom salts baths, and increasing her daily intake of green leafy veg. To my delight, she agreed to all three suggestions, and by the third consultation had noted a further improvement. She was able to do sport at school without using her bronchodilator inhaler. But she was still somewhat wheezy at night, despite implementing most of the anti-HDM measures most of the time. So it was time to discuss diet. You might imagine this would come up at the first consultation, and often it does, but one has to be tactical with teenagers; once Becky had seen some improvement, she was willing to consider further helpful actions, even if they were challenging.

Asthma can be a sensitivity reaction to foods, as well as to airborne allergens like HDM. By far the commonest foods implicated in asthma and eczema are milk and other dairy products. Andrea had mentioned at the first consultation that Becky had become a very colicky baby once she was weaned. She had been fine while she was being breastfed, which was for eight or nine months, but had started with tummy cramps, diarrhoea and accompanying screaming sessions once she started on formula milk. I asked if that was also when the childhood eczema had begun, and Andrea said yes, as a matter of fact, it was shortly after that.

"Does that mean I'm still allergic to milk?" Becky asked. "Have I got to give it up?"

The answer was: "We don't know yet. Let's Suck it and See."

An Elimination Diet

I asked Becky if she would be willing, just for two weeks, to give up **all** dairy products, namely milk, cream, yogurt, cheese, butter and any processed/packaged foods with dairy products in. Then she would note any improvements, and she would gradually reintroduce all the different types of dairy produce, one every

48 hours, observing and writing down any worsening of the wheezing, and any other symptoms. We wanted to see which dairy product(s), if any, were exacerbating her asthma. Some people are sensitive to milk but not to cheese, for example, and others are fine with any dairy products from goats and sheep but not from cows. So we were going to find out.

Becky stayed off dairy for two weeks, and then reintroduced a new food every two days, on the following schedule, which starts with the foods **least** likely to cause problems and ends with the most likely culprits. If any food she reintroduced did exacerbate the asthma, she was to wait till the symptoms had gone back to baseline before proceeding with the next food re-introduction. Here's the order we used, after 14 days off all dairy foods.

Day 1 – Goat's butter
Day 3 – Sheep's cheese
Day 5 – Goat's cheese
Day 7 – Sheep's yogurt
Day 9 – Goat's yogurt
Day 11 – Cow's butter
Day 13 – Goat's cream
Day 15 – Cow's cream
Day 17 – Goat's milk
Day 19 – Cow's cheese
Day 21 – Cow's yogurt
Day 23 – Cow's milk

Becky and Andrea had to be super-organised to make this work; it's a systematic process, and requires systematic planning and recording. You have to anticipate, pack lunches where necessary, and not end up at a pizza party unexpectedly. What Becky found was that she had no problems at all from any kind of butter, cream or cheese, and she was fine with goat's yogurt and sheep's yogurt. She thought she did get a slight increase in wheezing after the goat's milk, and Andrea agreed. After the cow's yogurt she definitely got worse, and drinking cow's milk set off an asthma attack, for which she needed to resort to a double dose of the bronchodilator inhaler. It also made her feel unexpectedly sick, although she had been drinking milk in tea without awareness of its effects, because she was having it every day. This process is called "unmasking".

The experiment Becky did is a modified version of the "Elimination and Re-introduction" method pioneered by the late great Dr John Mansfield, who in turn was taught by Dr Richard Mackarness. Its main result for Becky was that she now knew not only which foods to avoid (only three out of a possible twelve), but she also knew which foods she did **not** need to worry about, and could eat them freely. What a shame it would have been to have just said: "Stay off all dairy produce"; she would have missed out on lots of foods that turned out to be perfectly ok for her.

Everybody is different, and every body is different. Food allergies/intolerances are a form of physiological idiosyncrasy, and trying the kind of experiment that Becky did will give more accurate results than guessing. Nevertheless, there are some generalisations to be made. There does, clinically, seem to be a link between dairy products and asthma/eczema, and the common folk wisdom is that "milk creates mucus". Certainly many people, with or without asthma, report that milk (and in some cases other dairy products) give them catarrh, or mucus in the throat, or a blocked or runny nose. This is true, but asthma is not primarily about excess mucus, it is about bronchospasm.

Where an allergic reaction to a food is sparking off wheezing, the reaction is virtually always a response to the **protein** component of that food. Butter and cream are very low in protein, and didn't give Becky any problems. Milk, cheese and yogurt are higher in protein, but the nature of the protein depends on the species of animal. The main protein in milk is called casein. But cow casein and goat casein and sheep casein are all slightly different, and Becky's immune system could tell the difference (it is the immune system that produces allergic reactions). For her, sheep casein was fine, and so was goat's up to a point, but not in the form of milk. Cow casein was not ok for her as found in yogurt and especially in milk. But she was alright with cow's cheese. Why? We don't know for sure, but the ratio of protein-to-fat is higher in yogurt than in cheese; that's the most likely reason. We lose the specialised casein-digesting enzyme, rennin, from the stomach by the age of 6–8 years; nature only intended it for digesting breast milk. After that age we have to manage with pepsin and other general protein-digesting enzymes.

Could Becky's body have been reacting to the lactose in the goat's and cow's milk? Lactose is a sugar not a protein, but people can certainly react to it. It is not an either/or; it was probably a bit of both. Milk (of any species) is higher in lactose (milk sugar) than are yogurt, cheese, butter or cream. That's why humans have been turning milk into these products for 10,000 years; they are more digestible. Most people on the planet don't make the lactose-digesting enzyme, lactase. A few Caucasian people, mostly

Nordic types and some Indian people, can make lactase, and they are the only ones who can really drink milk without adverse reactions. But there may be long-term health effects for everyone, as noted in the paper "The Cow and the Coronary" published in the International Journal of Cardiology.[84] And finally, it should be remembered that lactose is sugar, and, as we have seen, overdosing on sugar isn't a good idea for anyone.

Becky continued to avoid milk and cow's-milk yogurt, she took her magnesium, and kept her room as free as possible of dust, HDM and moulds. When her parents saw how improved she was – she was off all inhalers by the time of our fifth consultation, thirteen months after the first one – they started doing a bit more dusting and vacuuming in the rest of the house, despite their busy commuter lifestyle. As Andrea remarked: "It's supposed to be parents yelling at teenagers to clean up their rooms, but with our family it's the other way round!"

Re-testing showed that Becky's magnesium level had normalised, so she was able to stop the supplement. Becky had one setback; she swam in a highly chlorinated indoor pool for half an hour, and that set off an asthma attack. She had to fish out her long-disused inhalers from the back of a drawer to deal with that, and it took two or three days to be fully better.

I said earlier that the food experiment Becky did was a modified version of an "Elimination and Reintroduction Diet". Let me explain how and why we modified it, and the drawbacks and imperfections of this method.

The "pure", original version of this method involves giving up almost all types of food for about ten days, subsisting on a diet of the very few foods that hardly ever cause allergic responses in anyone. "Lamb and Pears" was the first version, but we wouldn't use that now because pears now have too much sugar to be a mainstay of the diet for ten days. Modern versions would be something like lamb, salmon, turkey, courgettes, bean shoots, celery, olive oil, sea salt and mineral water. Then there would be the reintroduction phase, which is longer and far more logistically challenging than the initial ten-day period. Everything else the person normally eats would have to be added in systematically. Some practitioners add in one new food per day, some add in one per meal, and some add in one every two days, as I did with Becky. Some foods, like dairy products and grains, can take up to 48 hours to have their effect. Furthermore, in some diseases, especially arthritis, there can be a very long time lag between the food and its effect, making it hard to judge what's happening.

Some practitioners ask the patient to measure their pulse rate before and then 20 minutes after each food reintroduction; this, in addition to keeping a careful written record of any reactions, can also be a useful guide to which foods are a problem for that person.

The Elimination and Reintroduction Diet is an excellent way to unmask hidden food allergies, but if you have ever had a serious allergic reaction or anaphylaxis, then you must only ever do this under the close supervision of a clinician with the relevant experience and facilities to give adrenalin and so on. Practitioners can find more details about how to run an Elimination Diet in the book *Environmental Medicine in Clinical Practice* by Anthony, Birtwistle, Eaton and Maberly, obtainable from the British Society for Ecological Medicine, www.bsem.org.uk

In Becky's case, there were three reasons for doing only a modified version of the elimination and reintroduction process. First, doing the full version would have been far too difficult and demanding, and second, it isn't a good idea in a growing child; they need their calories! Thirdly, Becky wasn't ill enough to justify it.

On the other hand, there is a major disadvantage of setting it up the way I did for Becky. We **only** excluded and reintroduced dairy products, based on my educated guess – and Andrea's memory of Becky's childhood colic – that these foods were the most likely culprits. And we were lucky that we got clear results and identified the culprit foods, and that avoiding those foods helped get rid of the remains of Becky's asthma. BUT if Becky's trigger foods had happened to be, for example, wheat and/or corn and/or soya – all common allergens – we would have missed them. We would have got unclear results from our reintroductions, because she would still have been eating foods to which she was unknowingly intolerant. So there would have been no unmasking and no benefit.

So it is always a finely balanced decision, where food allergy/intolerance is suspected, whether to go the whole hog (excuse me) and do the full Elimination and Reintroduction Diet, or to do a modified version, or not to do it at all. Either way, it is far better to do this process under the guidance of an experienced nutritional practitioner. There are many potential pitfalls:

- The commonest error, on reintroducing a suspect food, is simply not eating enough of it. You do want to know if you have a problem with that food. You won't find out if you're intolerant to milk by having just one sip – you need to drink a whole glass. And of course, you would **never** try reintroducing a food to which you already know you react badly; the point of the exercise is to unmask intolerances to common foods that you are **unaware** of.

- Second pitfall: if the person is on medications to suppress their symptoms, again you may not get a clear response. Becky was in fact still on a low dose of inhalers when we did the dairy elimination-and-reintroduction experiment, but they were not controlling her asthma completely, so there was still enough wheezing going on to see the effects of food upon it.

- Third potential pitfall: compounding factors. Stuff happens, life intervenes. Some event other than the food you are reintroducing on a particular day can cause symptoms and muddy the waters. For instance, if Becky had gone swimming in that chlorinated pool on the same day she reintroduced butter, and she started wheezing badly, we might have concluded that she was allergic to butter. Wrong. She was allergic to chlorine. (Actually, that's not technically allergy. Chlorine is toxic to all of us. We don't know why it affects some of us more obviously than others, but it may be to do with iodine deficiency.)

- Fourth pitfall: the elimination-and reintroduction process only seems to work once, or at best twice. You can't keep repeating it unless you leave a gap of several years; you will get unclear results. So don't think of undertaking it unless you have cleared your diary and can really plan ahead.

Becky came back for a final consultation a year or so after the fifth one. She was fine, still off her inhalers, and playing netball. She had two questions, however. Firstly, the eczema had not quite gone. Now, everything I had done for Becky's asthma might well have dealt with the remnants of the eczema too, but skin problems can be stubborn. I checked her Vitamin E – important for skin health – and it was fine. So I referred her to a qualified medical herbalist (a member of the NIMH – National Institute of Medical Herbalists) who gave her a herbal cream. It cleared up the eczema within a month, which is unusually fast. Herbal medicine works brilliantly when all the nutritional and environmental factors have been dealt with. Indeed, most herbalists know this, and the person Becky saw would probably have put these basics in place had I not already done so.

Secondly, Becky wanted to get a kitten. She and Andrea wanted to know whether this would be ok; cat fur (and other animal furs) are a very common asthma trigger. If you have read this far you can guess my answer: Suck it and See. Not literally. I suggested Becky find a friend with a cat – she had plenty – and spend time cuddling the cat, and see how she got on. Face right in the fur – cat permitting – to be sure.

Becky tried this and she was fine. So she got her kitten and was very happy. She was lucky, but even asthmatics who are allergic to mammalian fur can still usually have a cat or dog if they observe these basic four precautions:

1 After stroking the cat or dog (or guinea pig/rabbit/gerbil/ hamster etc.), wash your hands instantly.

2 Brush the animal daily, then wash your hands. Or preferably get someone who isn't allergic to do the brushing.

3 Never let the pet into your bedroom. Ever.

4 Have a zero tolerance policy towards fur on the carpet/ furniture. Vacuum it up instantly. More housework – sorry!

Take-Home Tips For Autumn

◢ Pick wild blackberries.

◢ Pickle fruit and veg to last through the winter; it's what our great-grandparents did.

◢ Avoid mould exposure and house dust mites; keep your house/flat warm, but keep windows open. Let beds air, change pillows frequently, vacuum carpets, damp-dust exposed surfaces regularly.

◢ It's the start of a new term if you've got school-age kids. Take them for a dental check-up, but don't let the dentist put in metal amalgam fillings. These are at least 55 per cent mercury, and mercury is toxic to the brain. White fillings are probably safer. Good tooth-brushing and avoiding sugar are better still.

- Dental check-ups again: don't get fluoride drops or fluoride-containing fissure sealants. Fluoride damages bone, brain, thyroid, kidneys, ovaries and more. The dentist may not mention that she/he is using these; you need to request that she/he doesn't. Always ask the dentist what materials she/he is planning to put on/in your child's teeth. It is quite worrying how often dentists don't know the ingredients of substances they put in people's mouths every day, or the effects of those substances on the body at large. They have been told in dental school that it's all safe. There are countless published papers, from reputable sources, about the dangers of fluoride; hundreds are referenced in one book alone (Dr Paul Connett's *The Case Against Fluoride*), but your dentist may well not have read them.

- Avoid colds and flu – remember the first-aid package from the Winter chapter.

- Are you, or your elderly parent, taking prescription drugs, perhaps several? Early autumn is a great time of year to get them reviewed; you might not still need all of them. It's a good time because your GP has had a summer holiday.

CHAPTER 5

SEASONS OF YOUR LIFE

··

Staying Well at All Ages and Stages

This chapter is divided into five sections, all with case histories.

Pre-conception, Pregnancy, Birth And Breastfeeding

Pre-conception care

Our babies are affected by everything we eat, drink and breathe; before conception, in the womb and during breastfeeding. The quality of both egg and sperm is improved by good nutrition and damaged by exposure to toxins. So pre-conception care is the ultimate form of preventive medicine. We know now that our nutritional status has an effect not only on our own health but on the health of our children and grandchildren and generations beyond. And there is so much we can do to ensure the health of our babies.

Whatever substances are in a woman's body – the good, the bad and the ugly – most of them, including almost all drugs, will cross the placenta and get into the baby. If a woman is deficient in vital nutrients, there may be too little to nourish the baby properly, or even too little to conceive at all. On the other hand, the baby in the womb is very good at grabbing what it needs, so if a woman's level of iron, for example, is low or borderline at the start of pregnancy, she will be anaemic and exhausted by the end – all her remaining iron reserves will have gone into the baby, leaving her depleted. So for the health of the mother as well as the child, it makes sense to get levels of essential nutrients optimal before getting pregnant.

But these days we don't just have to worry about whether we've got enough of the good stuff – the nutrients. We also have to worry about the bad stuff, our "toxic load"; the synthetic chemicals that we have all absorbed from our polluted environment: air, water, food and soil. Throughout this book, but especially in Chapter 7, I discuss the sources and dangers of these toxins, and also how to avoid and "detox" them as far as possible. At no stage is this more crucial than before conceiving. Research has shown the very real risks to the foetus of toxic chemicals crossing the placenta from the mother.[85] This can be from either acute or chronic contamination. Acute contamination episodes, i.e. dramatic, one-off events, are better known, so let's start by briefly mentioning some examples; they may seem extreme, but although they are indeed extreme, they are sadly not irrelevant to us.

In the 1984 chemical disaster at Union Carbide's factory in Bhopal, India, babies died in the womb or were born with terrible deformities, and the damage continues to this day.[86] In Vietnam, 45 years after the end of the war, generations of children have been seriously disabled by the long-lasting effects of Agent Orange, a herbicide-plus-dioxin mixture that was sprayed on the jungle from 1962 to 1971. In Minamata Bay in Japan, a chemical factory discharged methyl mercury into the sea in the early 1950s, and people who ate the fish from those waters became ill with neurological diseases, and often died. Many babies were born dead or very disabled, and in many of those cases their mothers felt perfectly well during pregnancy – better than everyone around them, in fact – because all the mercury was going into the baby.

The UK is not immune. At least 16 babies were born with birth defects in the Northamptonshire town of Corby after the council had done reclamation work on land occupied by an old steelworks, between 1983 and 1997. The land was contaminated with numerous chemicals, which found their way into the surrounding area. After the out-of-court settlement reached in 2010, the case was compared to the Camelford disaster in Cornwall (see page 236), to the Thalidomide disaster, and to the Californian chemical contamination exposed by Erin Brockovich (as in the film of the same name), in which carcinogenic hexavalent chromium was dumped into the water supply of the town of Hinkley.

All these are instances of acute toxicity, however. What is more insidious, and far more common, is the "drip, drip" of low-level, chronic exposure to multiple unknown toxins. Tiny amounts, perhaps, but ongoing over decades. It is much harder, therefore, to connect cause and effect in any one particular case. We have known for many years about the damage that alcohol and cigarette smoke do to the unborn child. It turns out they are just the tip of the iceberg.

The placenta doesn't "know" what's toxic; it isn't "programmed" by evolution to expect any nasty artificial chemicals to be in the mother's bloodstream. It thinks everything there is food for the foetus, so in it all goes. The baby's blood circulation is really one with the mother's. An ironic result of this is that pregnancy itself can act as a "detox" for the mother – but not in a good way. If the mother is ill from excessive toxic load, she may well feel dramatically better by the end of her first pregnancy; she has "detoxed" a lot of her chemical contaminants through the placenta into the child. And it is the child who may then be very unwell. I have observed that the majority of sick children whom I see are first children; their younger siblings are usually fine. It seems that the oldest child received most of their mother's chemical load. For example, I see high mercury levels in the oldest child where the mother has a mouth full of metal amalgam fillings;

mercury goes in through the placenta. These are children with neurodevelopmental disorders; mercury is a known neuro-toxin.[87,88,89] But their younger brothers and sisters are usually fine; the first child took the hit for them.

This observation, by the way, is an example of what used to be called clinical experience, but is nowadays dismissed as "anecdotal evidence". There is no ethical way to test the hypothesis. I can't prove it; it is just what I have seen.

Pre-conception nutrition

So which are the most essential nutrients to get right before conceiving? Well, all of them really. But for healthy pregnancy I would single out vitamins D and E, all the B vitamins (that includes B12 and folic acid; most B complexes include the vital 400 µg of folic acid), the minerals zinc, iron, selenium, iodine and magne-sium, and the essential fatty acids (omega 3 and omega 6). I would follow all four golden rules on page 22 and also take a probiotic, especially if your bowel function is less than perfect.

If you take a prenatal supplement, i.e. a pregnancy multi-vit, check that it hasn't got added fillers and other junk in it (details in Chapter 6), and that any Vitamin D it contains is in the form of Vitamin D3, not D2 (your healthiest source of Vitamin D is, of course, sunshine on the skin – see Chapter 3). One of the prob-lems with multi-vits is that they often contain nutrients which compete with each other for absorption. For example, iron will stop zinc being absorbed in sufficient amounts, and calcium will inhibit the absorption of magnesium. So it's really better to take them separately if you are deficient, e.g. take iron at breakfast, zinc at dinner.

Pre-conception vitamins

Vitamin D is vital for the development of the baby's bones, teeth and brain. Deficiency of Vitamin D can cause all sorts of structural malformations. The main sources are sunshine and oily fish.

Vitamin E is essential for both male and female fertility, and for the proper utilisation of other nutrients such as Vitamin A, selenium and essential fatty acids. It's also needed for normal development of the foetal heart, and for speedier wound healing after abrasions and burns. It prevents oxidation of fats, i.e. it keeps them in the healthy form. Vitamin E is almost always low in men with low sperm counts and women with difficulty conceiving. Vitamin E is found in eggs, nuts, pumpkin seeds, sunflower seeds, tahini (sesame seed paste), wheatgerm, avocados, lettuce and good quality cold-pressed vegetable oils.

The B vitamins all work together, should be taken together as a B complex, and mostly occur together in foods, except for vitamin B12 about which more shortly. Let's look at them all briefly. Remember, the B vitamins are water-soluble. This means you can't store them, so you need some every day.

> **Vitamin B1 – Thiamine.** Like all the B vitamins, this is vital for the nervous system, and for processing carbohydrate foods and producing energy. Deficiency causes damage to the heart, muscles and nervous system. Deficiency also contributes to infertility, stillbirth and low birthweight babies. B1 is found in whole grains, pulses and red meat.

- **Vitamin B2 – Riboflavin.** Animal experiments have shown that lack of B2 leads to infertility, stillbirths and numerous deformities in the foetus, including cleft palate.[90] Supplement it together with all the other B vitamins, i.e. as a B complex. B2 is found in liver, meat, dairy products, some whole grains and leafy green veg.

- **Vitamin B3 – Niacin.** Again, lack of B3 may be associated with cleft palate and limb defects, probably because both B2 and B3 are essential for folic acid to work properly, and folic acid deficiency is associated with cleft lip and palate,[91] as well as with spina bifida (see below). B3 is found in meat, fish and dairy, and most whole grains but not maize (sweetcorn).

- **Vitamin B5 – Pantothenic acid.** Vital for the adrenal glands and central nervous system to work properly. Deficiency in pregnancy has been associated with many different abnormalities of the nervous system, and lack of B5 has also been linked with miscarriage in animal studies. Widely distributed in foods.

- **Vitamin B6 – Pyridoxine.** Essential to make RNA and DNA, the material that our genes/chromosomes are made of. Low levels in pregnancy are associated with a range of foetal abnormalities. Found in eggs, meat, fish, whole grains, nuts, seeds, avocados, bananas and most greens. Depleted by the contraceptive pill.

🌿 **Vitamin B9 – folic acid.** Spina bifida is a serious developmental condition where the bony spinal column fails to close around the spinal cord, leading to paralysis. It is definitively linked with deficiency of folic acid, as first shown by research published in 1980.[92] Now you might be thinking, "well, my mum never took folic acid supplements, and I don't have spina bifida." Ah, but your mum was probably getting enough folic acid from green leafy vegetables ("folic" as in foliage – leaves). The women in the studies were not.[93] However, I don't believe that this is the whole story with spina bifida. Its incidence varies greatly with geographical region, and significant differences occur even within a small area, which always indicates an environmental factor or factors. It has been found to occur with unusual frequency in mining areas in South Wales,[94] in a uranium-mining area in Zambia,[95] in the Shanxi province of China[96] and in mining areas in the Appalachian mountains.[97] So I suspect toxicity is in the mix along with folic acid deficiency; toxins are "anti-nutrients" (see page 272); they do their damage largely by destroying vital nutrients in the body.

🌿 **Vitamin B12 – Cobalamin.** Vitamin B12 is vital for the synthesis of DNA, RNA and red blood cells. Animal studies show that after a few generations of B12 deprivation there is an increase in the death rate of the newborns, as well as in the incidence of nervous system damage among the survivors. If you eat red meat, your B12 level will probably be ok, so the amount of B12 in an ordinary B complex should be enough to see you through a pregnancy. If you have tested low in B12, however, or if you are vegetarian or vegan, then the amount of B12 in a B complex is not enough to normalise your levels, and you need an actual B12 supplement, in addition to your B complex. B12 is a very safe substance; it is virtually impossible to overdose. The official "normal range" is set way too low, as explained in Chapter 6. I have called Vitamin B12 "Cobalamin", but it comes in at least four different forms: cyano-cobalamin is synthetic. Not the best. Yes, the "cyano" bit really is connected to cyanide! Hydroxy-cobalamin is a natural form, much better for you. Adenosyl cobalamin and methyl cobalamin are special forms, both of which the body should make from hydroxy-cobalamin, but this process doesn't work equally well in everyone. Some people have a genetic "glitch" affecting the biochemical pathways by which B12 is metabolised (processed) in the body. If you have had a miscarriage, or a baby with serious problems, or you are inexplicably failing to conceive, you can find out whether you (men or women) have this genetic glitch, by requesting a test called "Methylation report" from a company called Lifecode Gx. The test is very easy to do, but **not** easy to interpret; you'd need to find a nutritional practitioner who is able to do this for you. Lifecode Gx may be able to recommend a suitably qualified practitioner. The same thing applies to folic acid. Most people's bodies can utilise the ordinary folic acid that is found in green leafy veg or a B complex or a folic acid supplement. But a significant minority of people cannot, as we are now discovering through genetic testing. These people may need to take their folic acid as "methyl folate"; again, the genetic test above will tell you.

Whichever form of B12 you take, it should be as a lozenge to suck or a liquid to hold under the tongue, because it will be better absorbed from the mouth than it is from the stomach.

Vitamin B12 and folic acid work closely together with each other and with all the other B vitamins. Their biochemistry is interlinked, and they all depend on each other to carry out their many functions in the body; they're a team. So I wouldn't take any of them on their own except under the supervision of a qualified nutritional therapist or nutritional doctor (see Resources section on page 333). If you have been tested and found to be particularly low in one of them, you would normally be advised to take that one PLUS a B complex, but after a few weeks the B complex on its own should suffice.

The riboflavin (vitamin B2) in a B complex will turn your pee bright yellow. It's ok! It's just the body excreting what the cells can't use in that moment.

Finally, before we leave the B vitamins, a word about food sources of Vitamin B12. You will have heard that the best food source of vitamin B12 is liver. It is. But there is a question about whether pregnant women should eat liver. The concern is that liver is high in Vitamin A. While a good level of Vitamin A is vital for healthy pregnancy, Vitamin A deficiency is rare in the "developed" world, and excess may be more of a risk (especially if you take multi-vits). So I would say that it's good to eat liver occasionally, but not too often. And it MUST be organic, as the liver is the animal's detox organ, so if it's not from an organical-ly-reared animal it will be loaded with pesticides and antibiotics; not good for you, not good for the baby.

Pre-conception minerals

Zinc is absolutely essential for fertility and for healthy babies.[98] Both sperm and egg need it for normal development, and low levels during pregnancy have been associated with miscarriage, stillbirth and numerous abnormalities in surviving babies.[99] I almost invariably find zinc (and magnesium) levels low in chil-dren with hyperactivity, autism and other neurodevelopmental disorders.

Zinc plays a crucial role in pushing toxic metals such as nickel, mercury and cadmium out of the body. Conversely, the presence of those heavy metals can be a cause of zinc deficiency. Zinc is needed for hundreds of different enzymes in the body and for processing Vitamin A, and for the senses of smell and taste to work (kids with zinc deficiency are usually very fussy eaters). Zinc is used up rapidly in pregnancy, and I often find zinc deficiency in women who are trying and failing to conceive a second child soon after the first. Zinc is also used up rapidly by the contracep-tive pill, which depletes zinc and raises copper levels; this may be one of the reasons for "post-pill infertility". And I find zinc virtually always low in men with a low sperm count. Supplementing zinc is safe and easy, and strongly advised for both women and men trying to conceive and sustain a healthy pregnancy.

Zinc is found in seafood, and in meat, liver, eggs and root ginger. Also in nuts, seeds, pulses and some whole grains, but as explained in the Introduction, it may not be well absorbed from plant sources.

Iron is important for healthy pregnancy, although not quite as important as zinc. If you have plenty of energy and your muscles don't get tired after a day "on the go", and you never get short of breath, then you have enough iron reserves and don't need to supplement it. If you do get tired too easily, and your muscles ache and you get puffed out, please ask your GP to check your iron levels. NOT just your haemoglobin (Hb) levels; your actual iron, as measured by serum iron and Total Iron Binding Capacity (TIBC). Dividing iron level by TIBC gives the "Transferrin Saturation", which is a reasonable reflection of your iron reserves. The level of ferritin is even more accurate, but the GP may be reluctant because it is more expensive. Also, ferritin will be confusingly high if you have a cold or any other infection at the time of the blood test (ferritin behaves like an "inflammatory marker"), potentially giving false reassurance of normal iron levels.

A normal haemoglobin reading is not enough. Haemoglobin is the substance that our red blood cells are full of, and it carries oxygen around the body. Each molecule of haemoglobin contains an atom of iron, and if your iron is **very** low then haemoglobin will be low. But this test doesn't flag up the intermediate situation, where your iron reserves are low, but not low enough yet to impact on the actual level of haemoglobin. This is because the body is smart; it will use the last remaining iron reserves to make haemoglobin, so haemoglobin levels only fall once the iron levels are **really** low; this is iron-deficiency anaemia. You don't want to get to that point.

Iron supplements

Iron helps maintain energy supplies in other ways too; being part of the haemoglobin molecule is not its only job in the body. If you are iron-deficient, two important things to remember before you take an iron supplement:

1) The standard NHS supplement is ferrous sulphate, described by one of my patients as "industrial strength". Useful for a while if you are desperately anaemic, but most people find it extremely constipating. Look for ferrous fumarate, ferrous gluconate, ferrous citrate or, best of all, iron bisglycinate. They're all much gentler on the gut. Take at breakfast with Vitamin C and/or lemon juice to improve its absorption. Do NOT take it at the same time as zinc; save the zinc for dinner or bedtime.
2) If you are actually anaemic, it might not necessarily be due to iron deficiency; it could be due to deficiency of Vitamin B12 and/or folic acid. If so, taking iron will make things worse not better. So remind your GP – nicely – to please test for B12 and folate as well as iron.

Severe iron deficiency, to the extent of damaging the foetus, is uncommon in the Western world. Long-term vegan mothers with poor digestion may be at risk, however. The best food sources of iron are organ meats (liver, kidney, heart) and also muscle meat (ordinary meat) and egg yolk. It is also in green leafy veg, especially parsley and watercress, and to some extent in seafood, whole grains, pulses and nuts.

Selenium is a natural antioxidant, helping to fight both cancer and infections, and helping to maintain healthy chromosomes. It is vital for healthy conception,[100] partly via its role in the function of Glutathione Peroxidase, an antioxidant enzyme, and it is also an essential cofactor for the enzyme that converts thyroid hormone (T4) to its metabolically active form (T3). Selenium is necessary for normal growth and for pushing out toxins such as mercury, cadmium and fluoride. Men with low sperm count often turn out to have low selenium as well as low zinc, and I find that supplementing both can improve the sperm count within a few months. As a supplement, I find 100 micrograms of selenium daily is fine; it is possible to overdose if you take more than 200 micrograms a day (the standard dose) for long periods.

Selenium and Vitamin E work together to enhance fertility, so take them both. The best food source of selenium is Brazil nuts. Also other nuts, seeds and fish.

Iodine is vital to conception and healthy babies,[101] as has been known for over 100 years. We find iodine in any food that grows in or near the sea; mostly fish and seaweed. In the past, some babies born in areas where there was no iodine in the soil (always inland areas) suffered from severe mental and physical disabilities, owing largely to the poor thyroid function that results from severe iodine deficiency. These days our food comes from everywhere and anywhere, so there's a fair chance that some of it grew near the sea. So such extreme deficiencies due to low iodine intake may be less common, but there are now other factors making us low in iodine, namely the presence in our environment of the toxic halogens chlorine, bromine and fluoride.

You can check your iodine level by a simple urine test from Biolab (reception@biolab.co.uk) and you can take kelp or iodine supplements if needed, and eat seaweed and eat fish. Whether ordinary vegetables contain any iodine depends entirely on the iodine levels in the soil where they were grown, which is very hard to know. Sperm quality can often be improved by adding iodine to a man's diet, and it makes sense that the same would apply to the egg (ovum), although egg quality is of course far harder to test.

And the other minerals:

Magnesium. I have discussed magnesium a lot already; suffice it to say here that magnesium is essential for both egg and sperm, for healthy pregnancy, healthy baby AND for a safe and easy labour. Magnesium supplementation in pregnancy has been shown to reduce prematurity and admissions to the neonatal intensive care unit.[102] Low magnesium levels in pregnancy can make the contractions more painful than they need to be, and are linked to Pre-eclampsia,[103] a rise in blood pressure in the second half of pregnancy that endangers both mother and baby. In the emergency situation obstetricians often give intravenous magnesium, but it would be better to keep the magnesium levels healthy from the beginning of pregnancy, to avoid the emergency developing in the first place.

Magnesium is found in green leafy veg (again!), seafood, nuts, seeds, pulses and whole grains. Magnesium is depleted by alcohol and stress and diuretic drugs ("water tablets").

Chromium and manganese. Two trace elements needed in tiny amounts. Again, animal studies show problems in reproduction when they are lacking. If you test low, you can supplement with just one drop per day; Biocare make them in liquid versions which are well absorbed. They are (or should be) present in most prenatal multi-vits, but whether they are absorbed from them is another question.

Chromium is found in black pepper, liver, whole grains, cheese and many other foods. Manganese is in green leafy veg, whole grains, nuts and pulses.

Essential fatty acids (EFAS)

We need omega 3 and omega 6 EFAs, both for our general well-being and cell membranes and for making healthy babies with healthy brains. Controversy rages in academic circles about the correct ratio of omega 3 to omega 6 EFAs. The best we can say for sure is that we need some of each.

Omega 3 EFAs are basically components of fish oils, found in oily fish like mackerel, sardines, salmon, trout and herring. But there are vegetarian versions found in walnut oil and flax seed oil. In theory, the body can convert the vegetarian versions into EPA and DHA, the forms that our brains and cell membranes need, and which are found naturally ready-made in fish oils. In practice, what I find from blood testing is that very few people can make this conversion.

Dr Damien Downing points out that it is easy to overdose on fish oils.[104] Taking them for 3–4 months is beneficial – they are anti-inflammatory and good for the brain – but continuing for longer than that may be counter-productive. When I see children with ADHD, autism and other neurodevelopmental disorders, they have invariably been on fish oils for years. When I ask if it has helped, the answer is usually that it helped dramatically at first, but then it stopped helping after a few months. When it stops helping, it's time to stop taking it. Too much omega 3 will displace the equally vital omega 6.

Omega 6 EFAs are found in natural vegetable oils, of which hempseed oil is probably the best that you can use as food. Combine it with lemon or lime juice, raw garlic and a little honey to make a great salad dressing. As a supplement, evening primrose oil is the best; it's a great treatment for premenstrual syndrome as well as an aid to fertility.

Always take omega 3 (fish oil but NOT cod liver oil – too much Vitamin A) and omega 6 (evening primrose oil) at separate meals, to get maximum value out of them. And don't forget about olive oil, a valuable source of the omega 9 EFA, oleic acid. It's not a PUFA (poly-unsaturated fatty acid) like the omega 3s and 6s, it's a MUFA (mono-unsaturated fatty acid), and jolly good for us in numerous ways we are only just beginning to understand.

And one amino acid – Arginine. This bit is specifically for men. Several amino acids are important for sperm health, but there is one, arginine, which is especially useful for improving sperm count and quality, when used in conjunction with all the other nutrients mentioned above. Arginine is a component of many protein foods, but if sperm count or quality is poor, it's useful to take arginine in larger amounts, i.e. as a supplement. It is included in many multi-vits formulated for male fertility, although there are problems with multi-vits, as described on page 151 and in Chapter 6. But a word of warning; you shouldn't take arginine if you've ever suffered from genital herpes. It helps the virus replicate.

Avoiding chemical exposure

Alcohol and cigarettes damage the sperm, the egg and the baby. Ditto recreational/street drugs. If you would like to conceive and carry a healthy baby, Just Say No to them. Prescription drugs: stop them if possible, but obviously only in consultation with your GP. If you are on antidepressants you will need to withdraw very slowly. Allow time. The egg and sperm take about four months to mature. You want them to have done their maturing in a toxin-free, well-nourished body. So ideally you would start applying the nutritional and other guidelines in this section about a year before you intend to conceive. Let's say you begin in September by cutting out drinking, smoking, vaping and drugs, eating really well, getting nutritional levels tested, taking supplements if necessary and detoxing (Chapter 7) if needed. By March, chances are your body will have become a healthy environment in which the egg/sperm which will eventually make your baby can begin to mature. They will be ready by July; that's when you start trying.

All the above, although challenging, is fully under your control. What follows is only partially so.

The egg, the sperm and the foetus can all be damaged by the pollution that surrounds us.[105] In the city, our outdoor air is full of nitrogen dioxide, sulphur dioxide, benzene, polyaromatic hydrocarbons (PAHs) and numerous other toxic gases and particulates from petrol and diesel fumes, and from coal-burning and passive smoking. These poisons have already been implicated in miscarriage but also contribute to sub-fertility and to babies being born with health problems.[106] In the countryside, the pesticides sprayed on farmers' fields can cross the placenta.[107] They are EDCs (endocrine disrupting compounds) and are therefore bound to affect reproduction, which is controlled by the endocrine (hormone) system.

Weed-killer used on your own garden brings problems too. For example, the over-the-counter herbicide Roundup contains glyphosate, which is now classified as "probably carcinogenic to humans" by the International Agency for Research on Cancer (IARC), a branch of the World Health Organization (WHO). The IARC also point out, in their report of March 2015, that glyphosate is genotoxic, i.e. that it caused damage to DNA/chromosomes in human cells. It is potentially linked to non-Hodgkin lymphoma in humans, and convincingly linked to cancer in laboratory animals. A substance that is carcinogenic is also likely to be "teratogenic", i.e. to damage babies in the womb; the mechanism is the same: damage to our genes/chromosomes/DNA, which are the blueprint for life. (IARC reference coming up in Chapter 7.)

Similarly with the flea collar on your pet, or the drops you put on their fur to kill fleas – see safe alternatives on pages 110–112. Then there is the indoor pollution in our homes: cleaning chemicals, synthetic perfumes, fire retardants in soft furnishings, artificial toiletries in the bathroom, formaldehyde from chipboard furniture. There are heavy metals all around us and toxic fluoride in most toothpaste. Fluoride is added to your tap water if you live in the West Midlands, parts of north-east England or in the Republic of Ireland. And chlorine is added to tap water everywhere in the UK. It destroys the iodine that babies need. So does fluoride. Plenty about how to tackle all this in Chapter 7, but for now, here are some practical steps you can take to **minimise the risks at home**, especially in the year before trying to conceive:

⌀ Get a water filter, preferably a plumbed-in one rather than a counter-top jug filter.

⌀ Change to a fluoride-free toothpaste, such as those made by Green People, Urtekram, Kingfisher or Aloe-Dent. But still check the ingredients list, as some brands may start adding in fluoride to some of their products.

⌀ Let go of your synthetic perfumes, aftershave, deodorant, nail-varnish, hair dye, make-up. You can find safer natural alternatives for some of these in a good health-food shop, or you can learn to live without them. Many of my patients have, and feel better for it, as well as becoming more fertile.

⌀ Change your household cleaning products to safer versions, such as Suma or Ecover.

⌀ If you're a gardener, use organic gardening methods to control weeds without toxic herbicides. The birds and insects will appreciate it too!

⌀ For your cat or dog, use the safe methods of flea-control described in Chapter 3.

⌀ With regard to outdoor air pollution, there's really only one solution, and it's collective, not individual. Campaign, campaign, campaign. What's heating and choking the planet is choking us too, and seriously damaging our kids and our unborn babies.

Electro-Magnetic Radiation (EMR). This is another form of pollution that is physical rather than chemical, and it is equally harmful to the sperm, the egg and the foetus. Electromagnetic radiation is given off by mobile phones, mobile phone masts, cordless phone bases, wifi routers and 5G systems. Living near a pylon or electrified railway line is similar. Using a microwave oven ditto. There isn't space here to go into great depth about this; it would require another book in itself. But the key "take-home tips" are:

- Don't keep a switched-on mobile phone in your pocket. You will be irradiating your ovaries or testicles, and the egg or sperm that are trying to mature in there. If you are a man you will be lowering your sperm count.[108] Turn it off. Aeroplane mode is safe. If you are so busy and indispensable that you must be contactable at all times, at least carry it in a bag at a distance from your body.

- If you are – or might be – pregnant, don't put a laptop on your lap. Use a table. And don't sit close to the wifi router.

- Turn the wifi off at home whenever you're asleep or not using it. Or disconnect it permanently; you can still access the internet via an ethernet cable.

Both chemical toxicity and electromagnetic radiation can cause EPIGENETIC changes. That is, they can alter the way our genes function. That's how the damage they do can be transmitted to the next generation, and the next.

The ideal and the real

I'm aware that pre-conception care, as described above, is an ideal. And that, as the car bumper sticker says, the vast majority of people are caused by accidents. Some couples do come to me wanting to plan their babies in this way, and that's great. But most of the couples who consult me around this issue have, like Derek and Judy in the case history that follows, been struggling with infertility and/or miscarriage and/or stillbirth for some years already. Usually what works for them is putting into practice all the principles described above, plus one more important factor that we haven't yet mentioned: a trip to the sexual health clinic.

Sexual Health Clinics

Sexual health clinics are free, walk-in facilities, where both men and women can get tested and if necessary treated for STDs (sexually transmitted diseases). This is crucial, because undiagnosed genital infections can be a hidden cause of infertility. The clinic will check for chlamydia and other STDs that can lead to pelvic inflammatory disease and infertility in women, and it's vital that both partners get tested.

If the clinic wants to treat you with antibiotics, this is a time to say yes. You can do an intensive course of probiotics afterwards to help restore the good gut bacteria that will have been caught in the crossfire. If you've been trying for a baby without success longer than six months, it's time to visit the sexual health clinic, so infection can be ruled out or, if necessary, treated. It's also time to get a sperm count done.

Case History: Derek And Judy – Reversing Infertility

Derek and Judy were both aged 38. They had been trying for a baby for six years. They had conceived once during that time, but that pregnancy had ended in a miscarriage at 11 weeks. No one knew why, and the NHS will not investigate the causes of miscarriage until it has happened three times. That's three bereavements. They had, however, been through some fertility investigations. Judy had had ultrasound scans, hormone tests, and a "lap & dye"; that's laparoscopy (peeking into the pelvis through a cut made in the belly button), and hysterosalpingogram (injecting dye into the womb and fallopian tubes to check that there are no blockages). She was told that everything was normal; she was ovulating regularly, her hormone levels were all ok, her womb lining was fine and her anatomy was clear. There were apparently no obstacles to conception.

Derek had had a sperm test – just one, in six years of trying – and had been told:

"Well, it's a bit borderline, but nothing to worry about – it only takes one sperm to fertilise an egg, you know!"

Hmm. It only takes one, but the quality matters. The test Derek had done only told him the sperm count, percentage of "abnormal forms" and how motile they were. So all we really knew was that some of them appeared alright under the microscope and some of them could swim. We didn't know whether any of them could successfully fertilise an egg and lead to a sustainable pregnancy. Sperm quality has been implicated as a factor in miscarriage. The sperm count had been done four years previously, and needed repeating, as sperm quality can change over time.

I took a medical history, occupational/environmental history and food history from both of them. Judy had had post-viral fatigue for two years following glandular fever in her early 20s. She felt she had recovered, although she was still very tired in the evenings, but she put this down to her demanding job; she was a teacher in an inner-city secondary school, and cuts to school funding were making a hard job even more stressful.

Judy's diet was poor; a snatched bowl of sugary cereal for breakfast (all breakfast cereals are sugary), a sandwich from the staff canteen at lunchtime, and dinner was fish and chips or a takeaway curry, because she liked it and she was too tired to cook. Derek said he was completely well, but his diet was similar to Judy's, with the addition of 2–3 pints of beer most evenings, and 4–5 pints on Friday and Saturday nights. Sperm are very small, and they don't appreciate being pickled.

Even more significant was Derek's work; he was an electronic engineer, and had had several jobs that involved contact with heavy metals, including nickel, chromium VI, antimony and lead. He wasn't a welder, but he worked in a factory where he was not far away from people doing welding and metal-machining. He was also exposed to trichloroethane, a solvent used for cleaning the metals. He told me that the factory workers had to have blood tests every three months, but he didn't know what the tests were looking for.

At the first consultation we discussed what was possible in terms of dietary improvements. They both agreed to add an egg to their breakfast and take a box of salad to add to their lunch at work. They also agreed to cook and freeze some meals at the weekend, so they could have proper home-cooked meals, including vegetables, at least five evenings per week. I did blood tests for nutrients and toxins, arranged a repeat sperm test via Derek's GP, and saw them both six weeks later.

They had made the basic dietary changes, and Judy had noticed an improvement in her energy levels although she wasn't expecting it. The sperm test showed some deterioration from four years before; lower sperm count, an increased proportion of "abnormal forms" and slightly reduced motility. Judy's B vitamins showed up slightly low, but Derek's were very low; alcohol depletes the B vitamins and Vitamin C too. Both Judy and Derek were slightly low in a few minerals and vitamins D and E. These deficiencies were easy to correct, and I did so.

But Derek's toxicology tests showed up high levels of three out of the four heavy metals that he had worked with. When I told him this he went pale.

"I haven't got leukaemia, have I?" he asked.

"Goodness, no!" I replied. He was perfectly well in himself, and I had just seen a normal full blood count from his GP, so I could reassure him with confidence. "But why on earth do you ask that?"

"Because," he said, "my boss at work is off sick, and he's just been diagnosed with leukaemia, and they're saying it might be something to do with these heavy metals we use, and also the solvents."

Derek was clearly shaken; they both were. He decided there and then to look for a new job; in the same field, but in a much better-ventilated factory where his office and workshop would not be open-plan onto the area where welding and metal-machining took place. He managed this within a few months. It was a sideways move, not a promotion, but he decided that the air quality in his workplace was his priority, and said that he could feel the difference.

Getting Derek to cut back on his drinking was much harder. He wasn't addicted, but it was part of his culture, and he was very attached to his beer. I explained to him that not only was the alcohol probably damaging his sperm, but it also made it very difficult, if not impossible, to detox the heavy metals out of his system.

As well as repleting Derek's very depleted B vitamins, I wanted to get the accumulated toxic metals out of his body using Vitamin C, good minerals like zinc and magnesium, and all the detox modalities described in Chapter 7. But all of this relies on the liver being, as it were, available to help, and Derek's liver was busy every night detoxifying his alcohol, along with whatever herbicides and additives were in his (non-organic) beer.

Derek wavered, Judy's biological clock ticked on, and they did not conceive. Then, a few months after the second consultation, Derek decided to get a third sperm count done. It showed further deterioration. At that point, Derek confronted himself. His drinking wasn't interfering with his life but it just might, along with his occupational exposures, be interfering with his fertility. So he consulted the website Down Your Drink (www.downyourdrink. org.uk) which gave him a very helpful online programme to follow, to monitor and reduce his alcohol consumption. Down Your Drink does not advocate abstinence, only moderation, but Derek was an all-or-nothing person, and he chose after a few weeks of reducing his drinking to go "cold turkey". He found it very difficult, but he managed it.

He then came back to see me on his own, and I went through

with him the detox programme outlined in Chapter 7. Being the "all-or-nothing" type, he followed it almost to the letter. Retesting them both six months later, his heavy metals were gone, and his nutrient levels had normalised, as had Judy's.

Now the biological clock was ticking even louder. Ideally, one waits four months after getting the "all clear" (i.e. nutrient levels fine, toxins gone) before attempting to conceive, because that's how long it takes the egg and sperm cells to mature, and one wants them to be maturing in a clean, well-nourished environment. There is a slight risk, therefore, in conceiving part way through a nutrition and detox programme like this; a couple's biochemistry may be improved enough to conceive, but not yet improved enough to carry a pregnancy through to term. And I didn't want Judy and Derek to risk the trauma of another miscarriage. But of course this has to be weighed against the woman's age. Judy was 39 now, and they were simply not going to wait.

Interestingly, they did conceive exactly four months after that consultation with Derek, and nine months later Judy gave birth to a healthy baby boy. Interestingly also, Derek chose not to go back to his beer even though the situation was, as he put it, "job done!" This was partly because they were hoping to try for a second child, and also because, to his slight annoyance, he simply felt better off the booze, and had lost the beer belly that was beginning to appear when I first saw them.

So was this a case of male infertility (or subfertility to be more accurate), or both male and female? We can't be certain, and it takes two to tango, but my guess in this case is 80 per cent male, 20 per cent female. The male contribution to baby-making is somewhat neglected, which is a shame, as it is so much easier to test the sperm than the egg. That's why I've selected this particular case history for this section. Derek managed with NHS sperm tests, but for those who want more detailed sperm analysis, with a fuller interpretation, The Doctors Laboratory (TDL) in central London offers a very good and informative service through their Andrology department, although it is not cheap. Derek was not alone; sperm counts have declined dramatically in the Western world, falling by nearly 60 per cent between 1973 and 2011.[109]

Judy and Derek had been offered IVF, but had not wanted to go down that route except as a last resort. They felt it would have been quite an invasive procedure, and it didn't really make sense when all Judy's gynaecological testing had given normal results. Of the couples I see for fertility/preconception care, many have already tried IVF, which makes it harder to treat them. Of those who have not done IVF, about half manage to conceive naturally, like Judy and Derek, and about half do go on to use IVF. But interestingly, of the half who do go on to use IVF, most seem to succeed, and to succeed first time, and to suffer fewer side effects from the powerful hormonal treatments that are used. I think this is because we have normalised their nutrient levels, especially the zinc, which gets very depleted during IVF, so starting with optimal levels is of key importance.

I saw Judy twice more, during her pregnancy, to help maintain her nutrient levels and for an anticipatory discussion about breast-feeding. She breastfed successfully for over a year, and is now trying to tail it off (though her son disapproves!) in order to try for a second child.

Pregnancy

If you're already pregnant – congratulations! There's plenty you can do at this stage to enhance your health and that of your baby. You can't do an actual detox programme, but you can make every effort to avoid contact with environmental toxins, especially inside your home, as described above. You can and should follow all the nutritional guidelines described above. Taking a B complex is particularly helpful to reduce nausea in the early stages of pregnancy.

Listen to your body. Follow your cravings – up to a point. The exception is sugar. If you're craving sugar, you are probably low in one or more of the minerals that help to regulate blood sugar balance: zinc, magnesium, chromium and manganese. Taking these along with a B complex should help, as will eating frequently. The more often you eat – small, healthy meals or snacks – the less you will feel the urge for the sweet stuff.

Follow your aversions too; if you go right off a food you've previously enjoyed, so be it. I have one patient who found she suddenly hated white fish in pregnancy, even the smell of it, having previously liked it. Another patient developed an intense craving for celery, never having liked it before. The body moves in mysterious ways. So long as you are following the four golden rules on page 22 your body will usually tell you the truth; it mostly knows what it needs. I find that in women who've followed the pre-conception nutrition-and-detox protocol outlined above, there are far fewer troublesome pregnancy symptoms. But some degree of nausea in the early months is normal and harmless; find the moments in the day when you feel least sick, and eat the most nutritious foods you can in those "windows of opportunity". It will pass.

If you live in London, check out the Active Birth Centre, which has been empowering pregnant women to enjoy their pregnancies and prepare for the birth process for over 20 years. And if you want to read up about birth or breastfeeding, or indeed anything else, this is the time to do it. Make the most of your freedom; it won't last much longer! There are many excellent books, but I would particularly recommend the following authors: Sheila Kitzinger, Janet Balaskas, Yehudi Gordon, Ina May Gaskin and Michel Odent. An excellent book about breastfeeding is *Bestfeeding* by Mary Renfrew, Chloe Fisher and Suzanne Arms. I am mentioning it here rather than in the breastfeeding section that's coming up shortly, because once you are breastfeeding you may find it trickier than you expect to concentrate on a book.

Lastly, and contrary to standard practice, I would like to suggest: DON'T paint the nursery! For two reasons:

1 Most paints are toxic, especially gloss paints. You don't want to be inhaling those paint fumes while you're pregnant. As a compromise, it is possible to get less toxic brands, such as Auro, Ecos or Graphenstone, but still, if you must decorate, at least keep the windows open.

2 You Don't Actually Need a Nursery. Not yet. Newborn babies don't need their own room. In fact, the last thing they want is their own room. They've been curled up all warm and cosy for nine months, hearing your heartbeat, hearing your voice, in continuous unbroken physical contact. They need that physical contact to continue after birth; to feel securely held, next to a loving human being, most of the time. If they

are on their own in another room, **you** may know they are only a few steps away, but from their point of view you might as well be on Mars. They only know you're there if they can **feel** you there with them. They need to share your bed, as babies did for millennia (until the Victorians decided they knew better than nature) and as all other baby mammals do. You won't see new kittens or puppies anywhere but cuddled up with their mother. Evolution organised it that way to keep vulnerable young animals safe from predators and the weather. Your baby needs that too; that's her/his instinct, to be cuddled up safe and sound. Anything else naturally leads to terrified screaming, the signal that nature made to alert the parent to the baby's real and pressing need.

Bed-sharing works; it creates deeply confident, happy children, who become independent people sooner rather than later, and it also makes breastfeeding much, much easier.

Two good books about this are *Three in a Bed: The Benefits of Sleeping with your Baby* by Deborah Jackson, and *The Continuum Concept* by Jean Liedloff.

Birth

I'm not going to say much about the process of giving birth, as that would take a whole book in itself, and there are many good books about it already, as mentioned above. If you study them carefully, in good time, you can work out how to reduce your chances of being needlessly subjected to the "Intervention Cascade" that still goes on in many obstetric departments, even those which pay lip service to natural birth. But when you're actually in labour it is very hard to remember anything you've read, or anything you've written on your birth plan. You need someone else to be your advocate, to be there with you. And that person, whether parent or partner or friend, needs to have read whatever you have read, and to be familiar with your birth plan.

Before we get onto the "natural immunisation" that comes with breastfeeding, below, there is first of all the baby's encounter with the bacterial inhabitants of the vaginal canal. These help to prime the immune system of the baby's gut and respiratory tract, and protect against infection from unfriendly organisms. Babies who are born by Caesarean section miss out on these goodies, and sadly Caesarean sections are done more frequently than they should be.

Breastfeeding

Human babies need human milk. In an emergency, infant mammals can survive on the milk of another mammalian species. But, over millions of years, evolution has "designed" human milk as the perfect food for human babies. "Formula" is modified cow's milk, and cow's milk is for calves. Formula should be regarded as a drug; useful in emergencies, but with side effects,[110] some of them lifelong and serious.[111] Breastfeeding has tremendous benefits for both mother and baby. Let's start with the baby.

Benefits for the baby:

- Breastfed babies get far fewer infections,[112] and those that they do get are less serious than those of bottle-fed babies.

- Breastfed babies get less in the way of respiratory infections,[113] gastrointestinal infections,[114] urinary tract infections,[115] meningitis, ear infections[116,117] and many others.

- They also have fewer and less serious allergies, and a significantly reduced incidence of childhood cancer,[118] childhood diabetes, childhood obesity, SIDS (cot death),[119] enuresis (bedwetting), childhood asthma[120] and childhood Crohn's disease.[121]

- They have better mental development,[122] higher IQ[123] and fewer language impairments.[124,125]

- Those who were breastfed in infancy also have a reduced risk of many diseases in adulthood, including heart disease, cancer, obesity, osteoporosis, diabetes (both types), ulcerative colitis and Crohn's disease.

How does it work? There are probably many mechanisms by which breast milk protects babies.[126] Those we know about include the fact that human milk is full of IgA and other immunoglobulins (antibodies), plus leucocytes (white blood cells), anti-inflammatory factors and so on, which protect the baby directly and also stimulate the healthy development of the baby's own immune system. You could say that breastfeeding is the original natural immunisation. Formula can never successfully mimic this.

Benefits for the mother:

⬧ Mothers who breastfeed have a reduced risk of breast cancer,[127,128,129] endometrial cancer, ovarian cancer, osteoporosis, anaemia, rheumatoid arthritis[130] and anxiety.[131]

⬧ They lose weight more quickly after giving birth.

And quite apart from the health benefits, breastfeeding is simply easier and more convenient:

⬧ It's free.

⬧ The milk is always available, at the right temperature, in the right concentration and the right amount.

⬧ There are no feeds to make up, no bottles to sterilise, no wasted milk and no need to plan ahead.

⬧ Travel is easy, because of the above.

⬧ Night feeds can take place in bed; no need to go down to the kitchen.

⬧ The baby's poos are a lot less smelly!

Benefits for society:

⬧ A vast saving of NHS resources. Breastfed babies need far fewer visits to the doctor and far fewer prescriptions.[132,133]

BUT if breastfeeding is so wonderful, why doesn't every mother do it?

There are many obstacles placed in her way:

1 **Certain obstetric practices** can make it harder to breastfeed, for example giving pethidine late in labour (can make the baby too sleepy to feed), Caesarean section (can make it painful to sit up and feed), separation of mother and baby for any reason, well-meaning staff giving formula as a "top up" and lack of staff properly trained to assist with the establishment of breastfeeding.

2 **Undiagnosed problems** such as thrush of the nipples/thrush in the baby's mouth.

3 **Incorrectly treated problems** such as mastitis. Mastitis is an infection in the breast which can result from blocked milk ducts, which in turn can be caused by poor positioning while breastfeeding, by missing feeds or by wearing tight bras. The correct treatment for mastitis is in fact to feed as often as possible, to check the positioning of the baby at the breast, to have plenty of rest and fluids (as for flu), to use hot and cold compresses and herbal treatments, and if all else fails, antibiotics. But in any case, keep feeding!

4 **Incorrect positioning** of the baby at the breast can lead to "nipple sucking", which in turn leads to painful nipples and inadequate milk intake. The baby should have the whole areola in his/her mouth, not just the nipple. There can also

be incorrect positioning of the mother's arms, which can lead to blocked ducts, and there can be incorrect positioning of the mother in the chair; bad posture can lead to severe fatigue and backache. More detail on all this can be found in the book *Bestfeeding* mentioned above.

5 **Thinking the supply of breast milk is insufficient**. This is a very common mistake. Inadequate milk supply for a baby's needs is actually extremely rare. What more commonly happens is that the baby seems very hungry and wants to feed all the time, and the mother/grandmother/nurse/ midwife/health visitor misinterprets this as "not enough milk" or "milk not good enough". The solution is to let the baby feed as frequently and as long as she/he wants, and this may be far more hours of the day than the mother has been led to expect. With breastfeeding, demand stimulates supply; the more the baby suckles, the more milk will be produced. (With formula, suppliers create "demand".) Breast milk never runs out if the baby is allowed to suckle freely, "on demand", and the mother is well-nourished.

6 **Thinking the baby is underweight.** Many health professionals still use outdated infant weight-gain charts based on the growth of formula-fed babies, who put on weight faster than breastfed ones. This often leads to the recommendation to add some formula milk, which will then reduce the baby's demand for, and therefore the mother's supply of, breast milk, in a vicious circle. Hold your nerve and keep feeding; breast milk has kept our species alive for

millions of years. If it really ran out on a regular basis we wouldn't be here.

7 **Aggressive marketing of formula.** This includes free samples at GP surgeries, and adverts everywhere.

8 **Lack of support.** This can be moral, practical, professional or social support:
  - **Moral support** – every woman needs the backing and encouragement of family, friends and partner in order to breastfeed successfully.
  - **Practical support** – it helps immensely if someone else can take the older child(ren) out, cook the dinner or do the washing-up. I know this isn't always possible, but when it is it really makes a difference. Breastfeeding requires time.
  - **Professional support** – some women need help with breastfeeding technique and problem-solving in order to feed successfully. Not all women do it instinctively; some have to learn, and there are very few good teachers in this society. There are some, however, and the charity La Leche League is one of the best. Just because breastfeeding is natural and healthy does not mean it comes easily to everyone. We have very few role models; in pre-industrial times we would have watched our mothers, sisters, cousins and aunts breastfeeding, and it would have come automatically. It doesn't now, and there is absolutely no shame in asking for help. La Leche League can help, and some local branches of the

NCT (National Childbirth Trust) have breastfeeding counsellors who will come round. These sources of help are voluntary and free, and come from mothers who themselves have experience of breastfeeding. (Hospital midwives are rushed off their feet, and often don't have time to help, even when they do have the skills.)

- **Social support** – society at large and employers in particular need to become more supportive of breastfeeding. This is improving but needs to go much further. It should be totally normal to breastfeed in a shop, in a café, on a park bench, on the bus or train, in any public space. Every workplace should have a room where women can express milk for their babies, and it shouldn't be the toilet; you wouldn't prepare your own lunch in the loo – why should you have to prepare your baby's lunch there?

If you are the parent, partner, sister, brother or friend of someone who is breastfeeding and is struggling, here's how you can help:

- Turn up with dinner or cook dinner

- Wash the dishes

- Hold the baby while she has a shower

- Offer to call La Leche League or the NCT breastfeeding helpline for her if needed

- Remind her to sleep while the baby sleeps

- Don't suggest a top-up of formula. Remind her that she's setting the baby up for lifelong health, and it's worth it

- Pass her a glass of water – breastfeeding is thirsty work.

- Cook dinner again

Carrying your baby in a sling

A sling will keep your baby warm and happy, and leaves your hands free for household tasks or carrying shopping. It's natural and simple, and like co-sleeping, it gives babies the sense of security they need, as well as the sense of constant motion which they had in the womb. There are many good ones on the market, but my favourite is the Wilkinet. You should not have to put your hands under the sling/baby's bottom for support; that defeats the object.

You virtually never see a baby in a sling crying. But you often see and hear a baby in a pushchair crying, especially in the supermarket. Carry the baby in the sling and put the shopping in the pushchair. The shopping never cries.

One caveat, though. I have been horrified to discover that some slings now come with a handy little pocket for the parent's mobile phone. Don't put it in there, unless it's switched off or on aeroplane mode. The electromagnetic radiation given off by the phone would be an inch from the baby's heart. For that matter, please don't hold your phone anywhere near the baby's head or body. If the sling has a pocket, put paper tissues in there.

Childhood And Adolescence: A Survival Guide For Parents

Childhood

Keeping kids healthy these days is a challenge. They need space to run around and climb trees, but the urban outdoors is teeming with traffic; not safe, and filled with fumes that damage their lungs and their brains.[134,135] The indoors is full of screens and electronic devices which are inherently addictive, and stop them from playing, reading, sleeping and interacting with real people.

On the food front it is difficult too; sweets and junk food and junk drinks are everywhere, cleverly coloured and flavoured to be both attractive and addictive; what a shame they're toxic as well. You can't magic that commercial environment away; all you can do is strengthen your kids against it with the experience of good food, the information about what's in "bad" food and the knowledge that advertisers are deliberately targeting them so that food manufacturers can get rich at the expense of their health.

Let's start with the basics. If the only cold drink available at home is water, they will learn to drink water. If you install a plumbed-in water filter, the water will taste (and be) so much better that they'll actually want to drink it. But if there is fruit juice around they will go for that, for the sugar hit. Ditto squash/cordial/cola etc; these fizzy drinks are full of substances that belong in a chemistry lab, not in a child's body. Check their ingredients lists in the shop – and leave them there. But fizzy water is ok.

But what about "needing to have some in the house for when their friends come round"? Their friends will prove to be resilient and adaptable, and if there is no juice available they may even eat a piece of actual fruit. Kids eat and drink far more flexibly in other people's houses than in their own. They'll probably go home and demand that their parents buy whatever novel healthy food they tried at your house.

All the principles of healthy eating described in this book apply to kids as well as adults, particularly the four golden rules that begin on page 22. It can initially seem harder with kids; however much you whizz up that broccoli and hide it in pasta sauce, some kids will still spot it and refuse. But I have actually found that with many of the children I've treated, who have urgently needed to come right off sugar because it was messing with their guts and/or their brains, the process of retraining the taste buds from sweet to green is faster than with adults. The trick is that everybody in the household has to do it together. If you chuck out all the sugary stuff – cakes, biscuits, sweets, ice cream and so on – and have plenty of fresh fruit and veg around, and make it a family project, it may just be achievable. You can't expect little Johnny to abstain from sugar if Dad is munching doughnuts in the corner.

What children have told me is that they didn't realise till their parents instigated this project that carrots are sweet, red peppers are sweet, even onions are sweet. They couldn't taste that while they were still consuming the far more intensely sweet foods like cake and biscuits. It can take as little as two weeks for children's taste buds to adjust. If they will eat some greens – even cucumber is a good start – that also helps to shift the taste buds in the right direction. Psychologists have shown that it also helps to let children play with their food![136]

But sugar is powerfully addictive, and the craving for it is hard-wired into us, as described in the Introduction. So don't imagine that the process of weaning off sugar will ever be complete or perfect. When they encounter it, they will usually go for it, and the best and really the only thing you can do is to ensure that at least they hardly ever encounter it at home.

What to do when kids get ill? Most acute illnesses are viral, not bacterial, so antibiotics won't help them. Excessive antibiotic treatment is causing a major problem for the whole population by creating dangerous resistant bugs, bugs that no antibiotic can beat.[137] Excess antibiotics can cause more immediate problems for your child too, such as killing the friendly bacteria in the gut, leading to diarrhoea and tummy ache and sometimes long-term problems. We need to rediscover the lost art of nursing kids at home: rest, lots of water, lots of Vitamin C and some herbal remedies such as Echinacea (see first-aid package, pages 67–68). A few days off school will not ruin their education. I know it's hard to take time off work to nurse them, but that is a social/economic problem to which antibiotics are not the solution.

But if your child has an infection, how do you know that it is viral not bacterial? By persuading your GP to do what GPs always used to do: send a sample to the local pathology lab. A sample of sputum (phlegm) if it's a cough, a throat swab if it's a sore throat, a urine sample if it seems like cystitis, a poo sample if it's gastroenteritis. It only takes the hospital lab 48 hours to grow bacteria. During that 48-hour period you can use rest, water, Vitamin C, echinacea etc. as above (plus other specific remedies if it's cystitis – see Gwyneth's case history on pages 201–204).

When the results come back, if it **is** a bacterial infection, the lab will have tested to see which bacterium it is, and which antibiotic zaps that particular bug. So **if** your child isn't already better, then it's appropriate for them to take that antibiotic. This avoids taking a "best guess" or more harmful broad-spectrum antibiotic. And if the test comes back negative, i.e. no bacteria found, then you have avoided giving your child a totally needless antibiotic. If you do have to give antibiotics, follow them up with a course of probiotics to help restore the healthy gut flora (TTCs, as outlined in Chapter 2). There are plenty of child-friendly versions of probiotics (see Chapter 6).

What about prevention? Well, sorry to be boring, but fresh, home-cooked food, fresh air, exercise and plenty of sleep are the best way to keep kids well. "Do they need vitamin supplements?" is a question I'm often asked. Well, it depends. If they seem 100 per cent fine, probably not. If they're a bit under the weather and don't get enough sunshine, some Vitamin D3 drops through the winter would make sense. What about kids' multi-vits? Well, maybe, but Check the Label! If they're full of sugar and artificial flavourings and colourings, which many are, don't go near them. More info on this in Chapter 6.

What about chickenpox? Some kids sail through this with a few spots and no real illness. Others are covered in scabs and quite poorly – put them to bed. Liquid Vitamin E is very helpful here, to stop the spots from scarring; dab some on all the scabs frequently.

What about nits? Most kids catch headlice at school – nits are the eggs of the lice. Check out page 109 for how to deal with these safely and effectively; don't use over-the-counter lotions – they are insecticides and all insecticides are toxic and get absorbed through the skin of the scalp into the body and the brain.

Case History: Jason's ADHD

Jason was eight when his dad, Simon, brought him to see me. Jason had been diagnosed with attention deficit disorder, hyperactivity and dyslexia. He had "ants in his pants" big-time; he ran and jumped around the consulting room, interrupted constantly and couldn't settle to play any of the games his dad had brought with. He was also very bright and, at moments, charming.

He was getting into trouble at school because he couldn't sit still and focus. Jason certainly did have a problem, but so did the school. How reasonable is it to expect a bouncy small boy to sit still and focus on reading, writing and arithmetic all day long? It's not biologically natural. And indeed, Jason's dad told me that there were two situations in which Jason could in fact focus brilliantly. One was after a whole day of playing football. Jason did football courses in the school holidays, and at the end of a full day of football he was calm, relaxed, pleasant to be with and able to focus on whatever was necessary. He had run off the restlessness, as nature intended.

The other situation in which Jason could focus perfectly for long periods was playing with Lego. Because he loved Lego, and was astonishingly good at it. Simon showed me on his phone some photos of the towers and other constructions Jason had made, snapped quickly before Jason destroyed them; it was all about the process for him, not the outcome. He could focus on doing Lego simply because he loved it, and had chosen to do it, and He Was Not Bored. Children with ADHD have zero tolerance for boredom, and Jason found the three Rs boring. He did need some help, but there is also a problem with an education system that expects kids to tolerate boredom; education should be entertaining, especially in the early years, and for kids like Jason, the day needs to start with sport – lots of it.

Jason's diet diary was frankly terrible. Packaged cereal (full of sugar), sausages, chips, burgers, ice cream, crisps, sweets and fizzy drinks. Not a vegetable or a piece of fruit in sight, no healthy fats (which the brain needs) but plenty of bad ones, not enough real protein, and all the carbohydrate was refined, not whole grain. Sugar and additives galore.

Some delicate questioning elicited the fact that Jason's dad's diet was pretty similar.

"But my wife Sarah, she's into all this healthy eating business – she has fruit and veg and even avocados, brown rice and whatnot. But me and Jason we don't go for that stuff, do we?" He winked conspiratorially at Jason.

"But you have, um, ah, you have come to see a nutritional doctor. Were you not expecting any eating changes?"

"We thought you could give him blood tests and supplements."

Ah. Well, I don't like to do blood tests on small children unless it's really, really necessary. And it wasn't with Jason; 20 years of working with such children told me he would be low in the B vitamins, Vitamin D, zinc, magnesium and the omega 3 and 6 essential fatty acids. And he needed to start eating real food rather than taking supplements, at least initially. But to my surprise, Jason himself wanted the blood tests.

"I'm never gonna eat anything green, ever," he said, "unless you can **prove** to me that I need to." I told you he was bright. (Many children with ADHD and dyslexia are very gifted, but not necessarily in the areas which our narrow National Curriculum values most highly. Seventy-five per cent of students at the prestigious St Martin's School of Art have dyslexia.)

Fortunately, the nurses at Biolab, where I saw Jason, are used to taking blood from children, and they use a local anaesthetic cream to make it completely painless. I had one more attempt at dissuading Jason and Simon from spending money on tests, but they were both adamant.

Luckily, Sarah took a day off work to come with them to the second consultation. The test results were as predicted. Jason wanted "vitamin drops like my cousin has, and to keep eating what I like." I wanted Jason to eat fruit and veg, organic meat and fish and eggs, potatoes, whole-grain pasta, rice – just ordinary real food without additives and sugar. His mum, Sarah, had been trying for over a year to get Jason (and Simon) to eat properly, so what I was advising wasn't new or radical. But the test results seemed to make all the difference.

"Alright," said Jason, "I'll try eating all that healthy stuff. But not vegetables."

At a follow-up appointment three months later, Jason was eating much better, and both his parents and his teacher had noticed that he was calmer.

"But he still won't eat veg," said Sarah. "Now we've thrown out the sweet stuff he is eating four or five pieces of fruit a day. Is that ok?"

Well, these things are relative. Ideally, one would want Jason to eat a lot of veg and a bit less fruit, for reasons already explained. But compared to how Jason was eating before, all that fruit was wonderful.

At this point I did indeed give Jason some supplements, in

liquid form, of the nutrients he had been lacking, including both omega 3 and omega 6 essential fatty acids (EFAs), for a while. (More on omega 3 and omega 6 EFAs in the Appendix – of the book, not the body!) Probably because of the zinc drops, his taste buds tuned up, and he started eating the occasional bit of courgette, red pepper and carrot. To get him to eat actual greens, though, we resorted unashamedly to bribery. One portion of broccoli meant 50p in the pot towards more Lego. So greens with dinner every night for two weeks meant £7.00 towards new Lego kit; it worked.

Jason continued to become calmer – greens contain magnesium and magnesium calms people down – but he would occasionally have a junk and sugar binge at a friend's birthday party, and then he would become completely unmanageable for a day or two. But he was a smart kid, and eventually saw the connection himself, and began to exercise some restraint.

Jason's reading ability also improved. Two reasons for the improvement: one, the Vitamin D, B vitamins, essential fatty acids and other nutrients helped the neural circuitry in his brain to work better, and two, his increased calmness meant he could now focus even on tasks he disliked, such as learning to read. So he began to be able to do what dyslexic children need to do in order to become fluent readers, namely to work very hard at it. It just wasn't possible before.

Within a year, Jason's teacher was noting a marked improvement in his schoolwork. He could pay attention, and his reading age had shot up, although his spelling was still atrocious – you can't have everything. But his teacher did complain that although his focus was better, he still fidgeted (as hyperactive children do) and he was always fiddling with something during the lesson.

"But I NEED to fidget!" Jason told me. "I actually can concentrate better when I fidget!"

He was absolutely right. It still wasn't natural for him to sit still; he needed to move his body. I wrote to the school and suggested that Jason be not just allowed to fidget but actively encouraged to fidget. I asked Sarah and Simon to get him a squidgy "stress ball" to squeeze and play with during lessons, and to ask the teachers to let him jiggle his feet under the table if he needed to. And I also asked Simon if instead of driving Jason to school he could walk him there.

"But it's a half-hour walk!" said Simon.

"Good," I said. "He'll be calm and focused when he gets there."

"Yes, but then I've got to walk half an hour back home!" Simon protested.

In the end they both got scooters, and zoomed along the pavement to school. The school had a shed in the playground where Jason could park his scooter. Jason got happier and calmer, and Simon got fit.

At our final consultation, Jason was doing very well, and Sarah told me that she had joined the Board of Governors of his school, and was trying to persuade them to teach cookery and gardening to the kids.

"We don't have a garden at home, we live in a flat, but I think if Jason could learn a bit about growing food himself, as well as cooking it – well, it would make so much difference. And it's physical, not classroom-based. I know he'd enjoy it and really benefit; all the kids would."

Amen to that. And good luck, Sarah. Kids need to learn gardening at primary school, and horticulture should be a GCSE subject at secondary schools. Why not? (They already do "Food Tech" – although why that can't just be "Cookery" beats me.)

Adolescence

The hazardous environment faced by today's teenagers is unprecedented; everything listed on page 186 in relation to children applies to teens too, plus there's alcohol, tobacco, cannabis of various degrees and the hard-drug dealer at the school gate. And social media and online pornography. And the pressure to be ridiculously, impossibly beautiful according to someone else's commercial, unnatural idea of what beauty is. And the knowledge that they are facing ecological catastrophe and economic collapse: that they may never have a steady job or own their own home. That their planet is becoming uninhabitable. They know. Consciously or unconsciously, they know more deeply than their parents can what it is that they are facing. So it's no wonder that some of them seek refuge in the oblivion of assorted dangerous substances. All you can do is be there, support them, listen well and keep breathing. And try to find that impossible balance between cutting them some slack and trying to keep them safe. For now, a parent's place is in the wrong. But – this too will pass.

And now, down to earth with a case history about something that really bothers teenagers – acne.

Case History: Maya's Acne

Maya was 16 and gorgeous, but her face was covered in spots, erupting in various stages of red and yellow unpleasantness. Her GP had tried tetracyclines – powerful broad-spectrum antibiotics – but they gave her severe diarrhoea. Then he had tried putting her on the contraceptive pill, but it gave her mood swings and depression; it does that to some people. Finally, he wanted to try Roaccutane, but Maya's mother had read up about the long-term side effects of Roaccutane and put her foot down. So she brought Maya to see me.

Teenagers in current Stone Age tribal societies tend not to get acne. Teenagers in tropical rural villages tend not to get acne. So it can't just be hormones; it has to be some nutritional and/or environmental factors, some things about the way we live now, that **combine** with the hormonal changes of adolescence to make their skin (not to mention their brains) erupt in a flaming mess. Acne is to do with excessive secretion of sebum, or grease, onto the skin. In identical twins, the secretion of sebum is the same, i.e. it's genetic, but the degree of acne that results is very different between the identical twins, which suggests environmental factors at play.[138]

I suspect that air pollution is a factor, ditto lack of sunlight, and in some teenagers, especially girls, nickel sensitivity contributes. (Nickel is in stainless steel, so cheap earrings and other piercings are a possible source, as are orthodontic devices; more on this in Chapter 7). But mostly, predictably, as you've probably guessed by now, it seems to be connected with the gut. If you can clear the gut and restore a healthy population of the TTCs (good gut bugs; see Chapter 2), you can clear the skin. Eventually.

Maya was a bit of a chocaholic, by her own admission, and she was a fruit-a-holic too. Her breakfast and evening meal were fine, but in a futile and quite unnecessary attempt to lose weight, she was skipping lunch. Instead, she was eating lots of ready-made fruit salads from the supermarket, mostly melon and grapes, which are high in sugar, so would be feeding the unfriendly bugs in the skin and the gut. And she had no idea that those conveniently pre-chopped chunks of fruit in their plastic packaging had been sprayed with synthetic chemicals to keep them looking artificially fresh, when they were in fact several days old. And that those chemicals do not have to appear on the label. I didn't know either, till I read Joanna Blythman.[139]

A stool test showed an overgrowth of yeasts (single-celled fungi) and unfriendly bacteria in Maya's intestine, even though she had no abdominal symptoms. A urine test showed vanishingly low iodine (for probable reasons why, see page 75) and a blood test showed slightly low Vitamin D and very low zinc. The low zinc level may have been a result of the disease process rather than a cause; an inflammatory process like acne will use up a person's zinc very quickly, leaving less of it available for tissue healing, repair and growth.

First, we had to stop Maya feeding sugar to the unfriendly bacteria and yeasts. She agreed to wean herself off the high-sugar chocolate she was eating, by shifting gradually from 50% to 60% to 70% and finally to 85% dark chocolate. She found it much harder to let go of her fruity snacks, but I persuaded her to have a proper lunch instead, and she agreed. Interestingly, deprived of her fruit fix, she developed a rather helpful craving for salad. Salad contains all the same super-healthy antioxidants as fruit does, but without the sugar (and, in Maya's case, without the chemical preservative glaze on the pre-packaged fruit salads).

I gave Maya a lot of probiotics (good bacteria) for her gut, and herbs to reduce the numbers of the unfriendly bugs. (For which herbs, see page 91.) I also gave her Vitamin D, zinc, lots of Vitamin C and lots of iodine. And I warned her to hold her nerve; the gut gets repaired before the skin does, and the skin may get worse before it gets better.

It did. Maya was a determined young woman and she was also desperate. She stuck to her supplements and her salads and her sugar-free regime and she endured a month of even worse acne. Then slowly her skin started to improve. Within three months it was visibly better. Within six months it was almost clear, and within a year you wouldn't have known she had had acne. There were no scars because I got her to put Vitamin E oil on the spots as they started to scab over.

As Chinese medicine has known for thousands of years, what happens in the skin reflects what's happening in the gut. When the type of regime described above does not clear the acne completely, as it did for Maya, I would refer the young person on to a herbalist registered with the NIMH, for herbals creams and possibly oral herbal remedies as well, to complete the task.

Young Adulthood, 18–35: A Few Tips On The Wing

Most people in this age bracket are fairly fit and well, and/or too busy to think about their health much. This is the stage where many people, especially men, appear to be able to get away with eating badly and drinking too much and smoking – but it will start to catch up with them later on. So this is the age at which to put good habits in place; read the Introduction and the relevant seasonal chapter, and do whatever you can to eat well and sleep well and exercise a lot. It's preventive medicine. Because if you think you're busy now – wait till you have kids.

Case History: Elsa's Period Problems

Elsa was 28, and suffering from severe period pains that laid her low for nearly a week out of every month. She struggled into work sometimes; other times she had to stay in bed and call in sick. She also had quite bad pre-menstrual syndrome, or PMS. In the 7–10 days before her period began, she had sore breasts, sugar cravings and irritability; she would snap at her friends for no reason, or burst into tears at the slightest thing. It was all making her life miserable and difficult.

Elsa's diet was alright – ish. She wasn't eating any "bad" foods but there were a lot of good foods missing. In particular, she wasn't eating any of the foods that contain Vitamin E, which is essential for a healthy menstrual cycle. So I suggested she add eggs, avocados, nuts, seeds (sunflower and pumpkin seeds) and lettuce to her diet.

I also gave her supplements of Vitamin E and of the other nutrients that help in this situation: Vitamin B6 together with a B complex, magnesium (to help the womb muscles relax and release the menstrual flow) and evening primrose oil. All of this helped, but not quite as much as I expected. There was something else going on.

At our second consultation I went into more detail about possible sources of toxicity. It turned out that Elsa constantly drank water out of plastic bottles which she left in the car – so the sun warmed them up through the windows – or on a shelf above a radiator at home. She also wrapped all her leftover food in clingfilm or similar plastic wrap. Lastly, she worked in a shop, where she handled the till-roll all the time. Most till-rolls contain BisPhenol A (BPA), a toxic plastic chemical, and it goes into the body through the skin. So Elsa had at least three sources of exposure to plasticiser chemicals such as phthalates and BPA. These toxins actually showed up in a very specialised lab test to which I had access at the time I saw Elsa, but even if we hadn't been able to do the test, the history was clear enough.

These plasticiser chemicals are, like insecticides and other biocides, **oestrogen mimics**. They are a type of EDC – endocrine-disrupting compound. The endocrine system is the hormone system, and Elsa's was certainly disrupted. Her GP had done tests which showed that her oestrogen and progesterone levels were normal. But oestrogen mimics such as plasticisers and pesticides sit on the molecular receptors that oestrogen is supposed to sit on, thereby having similar effects to oestrogen and progesterone, but more so.

Detoxifying these chemicals out of the system is possible, but not easy. Firstly, Elsa had to stop putting them into her body. She had to start carrying her water in glass bottles, not plastic. You can buy these with a padded cover, or buy the cover separately in a camping shop, to protect them from breakage. Second, she had to stop wrapping food in plastic wrap – this is so thin and soft that its plasticiser chemicals leach into everything it touches. And she had to NOT replace it with aluminium foil because aluminium is toxic too – sorry! So she simply put leftover food between two plates in the fridge, and carried snacks to work in a brown paper bag (they still exist) just like her grandmother used to do.

Thirdly, there was the problem of the till-roll in the shop. Luckily it is possible to get BPA-free till-roll; many health-food shops use it. Eventually, after much explanation, Elsa's boss, the shop manager, was persuaded to buy some of this, from the Green Stationery Company; perhaps he worked out that it would be helpful to him if Elsa was not off sick so much. (The EU is going to ban BPA in till-rolls from 2020, but at time of writing it is not possible to know what impact, if any, that will have on the UK.)

Detoxing the EDCs out of Elsa's body involved saunas, done as described in Chapter 7, and taking Phosphatidyl Choline as well as her other supplements. A year after her first consultation she reported herself 80 per cent better, and very happy. And when she has kids, she won't wrap their food in plastic, or give them drinks out of plastic bottles. Plastic is toxic to us directly, as well as via being toxic to the planet.

Case History: Gwyneth's Cystitis

Gwyneth came to see me because of recurrent cystitis. Cystitis means a painful bladder and frequent painful urination, and feeling a strong urge to pee even when the bladder is empty. Gwyneth was 24, in a steady relationship, and she got cystitis every time she had sex and quite often when she didn't. There was no problem with lubrication and she was happy with her boyfriend.

Each time she got cystitis, her GP gave her a course of antibiotics (without first sending off a urine sample for testing), and she then got thrush (a vaginal infection with the yeast Candida albicans). Many women are caught on this merry-go-round, and it isn't merry. The antibiotics kill the good bacteria in the vagina as well as the gut, and then fungal organisms such as Candida albicans, always present in small numbers, jump into the breach and multiply wildly. Then Gwyneth would go back to her GP and get anti-fungal pessaries, and the thrush would go away, but soon the whole cycle would start again.

The first approach to prevention was, of course, to make sure Gwyneth was drinking plenty of water. The next thing was to make sure she asked her GP to send a urine sample to the hospital lab next time she got cystitis, which he duly did, and agreed to hold off on the antibiotics. While she was waiting for those test results, I gave Gwyneth all the standard natural remedies for cystitis: cranberry (concentrated in a tablet, NOT cranberry juice, because that has added sugar), the herbal remedy Uva Ursi (bear-berry), fresh parsley made into a tea with boiling water, D-mannose[140] and some potassium citrate to alkalinise the urine.

Four days later Gwyneth's symptoms had completely resolved, and she got the test results from the GP – no infection! No bacteria grown from her urine sample. A couple of white blood cells were found, indicating a degree of inflammation, but inflammation is not always due to infection; it can result from anything that is irritating the bladder. The GP shrugged, and agreed that antibiotics were not needed.

A longer-than-usual time elapsed before Gwyneth got cystitis again, and the same thing happened; she sent a sample off, and it came back negative – no bugs – by which time the natural remedies above had got rid of her cystitis symptoms. This was encouraging but a little mysterious; what was causing Gwyneth's symptoms, if there was no infection present? And anyway we didn't just want to treat it, we wanted to prevent it happening again.

Gwyneth's problem seemed like Interstitial Cystitis, a condition in which the bladder lining is inflamed but no infective organism is found. It could be that there is an organism there, perhaps viral or fungal, that refuses to grow in the lab or just isn't looked for. Or it could be that something quite other than infection is irritating the bladder lining and causing it to become inflamed. That can occasionally be a food causing an allergic reaction – I have seen this several times, where people have done a full elimination diet protocol (see page 135) and identified one or two foods to which the bladder lining reacts – or it can be an indirect reaction to dysbiosis in the gut (see page 83). In that case, unfriendly bugs in the gut are producing metabolites (waste products) which are absorbed into the bloodstream, and pass from there into the bladder, which doesn't like them, and becomes inflamed and sore, resulting in the classic cystitis symptoms of having to rush to the loo all the time, but peeing only small amounts and painfully.

Was that the case with Gwyneth? We didn't know. She had no gut symptoms, but people can have dysbiosis without gut symptoms. And as a penniless Master's student with debt accumulating, Gwyneth wasn't about to embark on an expensive stool test. However, after so many courses of antibiotics, Gwyneth certainly needed a course of probiotics, and I gave her some.

In the end, Gwyneth herself came up with a theory. She wondered if her bouts of "cystitis" coincided with her occasional evenings of drinking rather large volumes of very cheap red wine with her boyfriend. It was an easy theory to test. She stayed off the wine for a few weeks, during which time she had sex several times, without getting an attack of cystitis. Then she spent an evening drinking her favourite cheap plonk – and the next morning the cystitis was back, full throttle. She now knew what to do to get rid of it, and didn't even bother getting tested for infection this time.

Gwyneth had found the cause and the solution herself, which often happens once people start thinking in terms of cause and effect, and observing themselves and their reactions more closely. She decided that prevention was better than cure, and abandoned the cheap red wine. She is able to drink other alcoholic drinks, in moderation, without getting cystitis, and she does so occasionally.

It probably wasn't just the alcohol. It was probably the combination of alcohol, dehydration, and all the sugar, pesticides, sulphur dioxide and other rubbish that is found in cheap vino. Gwyneth doesn't get cystitis any more, and is slightly less penniless now she has almost stopped drinking.

The Dawn Of Middle Age, 35–50

You can't get away with that mad lifestyle any longer. Nature won't let you. If you are rushing around like crazy, not making time to cook, if you are drinking and smoking and sitting in your car, not exercising and also not making time to "stand and stare", something's gonna give.

I see a lot of people between the age of 35 and 50 who ask me, "But why should I have got ill **now**? I've been living like this for 15 years!" Exactly.

Case History: Rajiv's Diabetes

Rajiv was 42 and in shock. He had just been told by his local hospital in Paris that he had developed type 2 diabetes. It had not, however, come completely out of the blue; his blood sugars had been in the "pre-diabetic" warning range for a couple of years. He hadn't ignored that; he had worried about it, and had tried unsuccessfully to lose some weight. Now the hospital had offered him the drug Metformin to lower his blood sugar levels. He had tried the Metformin, and it had lowered his blood sugar levels, but he didn't feel good on it; he felt nauseous and had gut ache and a strange taste in his mouth.

He wanted to try a more natural approach, but his lifestyle was anything but natural. He worked internationally as a management consultant, so he was constantly travelling, staying in hotels, and not in charge of his own meals. He brought me two one-week food diaries, one at home and one while away working. The "at home" one had regular meals and not too much sweet stuff, but apparently it only accounted for about one week in four. The "away" food diary, which Rajiv had recorded with meticulous precision, was full of both sweet and savoury junk-food snacks, grabbed on the run, often in airports, at all hours of the day, between work commitments. And remember, even "savoury" processed food snacks usually contain a lot of sugar. Both food diaries showed two major, connected problems. He was drinking masses of milk, about one-and-a-half pints a day (0.86 litres), and he was eating no eggs, fish or meat. This latter was a religious tradition and was non-negotiable.

So here was my dilemma: to get Rajiv's blood sugar levels down, he needed not only to cut out sugar, but also to cut out all refined carbohydrate (white rice, white bread, white pasta etc.), because it breaks down rapidly into sugar in the gut, causing in turn a rapid rise of sugar level in the blood. He even needed to reduce whole carbohydrates such as brown rice and root vegetables to quite low levels. His main food sources needed to be instead protein and good fats. That would ideally mean animal foods. But the only animal food Rajiv was consuming – milk – was problematic because it is full of lactose, and lactose is a sugar composed of two smaller sugar molecules, galactose and, yes, glucose. **Not** what a diabetic needs.

So we did what we could. Rajiv agreed to cut out the milk and replace it with organic cheese, yogurt, cream and ghee (clarified butter). All of those are very low in sugar, and full of good fats (ghee and cream and cheese) and protein (cheese and yogurt). He also agreed to eat much more vegan protein – pulses like chickpeas, beans and lentils, plus nuts and seeds. The pulses are a mixed blessing because they contain as much carbohydrate as protein, but at least it is whole carbohydrate, and they are full of fibre, which helpfully slows down the absorption of sugar (from the digestive breakdown of carbohydrate) into the bloodstream. Nuts and seeds are mostly protein and fibre and healthy fats. Fortunately Rajiv was able to digest all these foods without excess gas production; not everyone can!

BUT all these changes could only be made when Rajiv was at home. For the 75 per cent of the time he was travelling for work, his diet remained almost as appalling as before. I wondered aloud why the hotels where he stayed could not provide proper food for him.

"Because they don't cater for strict vegetarians," he explained.

Unsurprisingly, as Rajiv was a frequent flyer, his level of the toxic metal nickel was excessive (see nickel in aerotoxic syndrome, pages 263–270). Nickel interferes with glucose metabolism,[141,142] and pushes out vital minerals like zinc which are necessary for insulin production. So I gave Rajiv the missing minerals, and Vitamin C and methionine to try and detox the nickel. (Methionine is an amino acid that helps remove nickel.) But of course he kept "retoxing" himself with the frequent flying. I also gave Rajiv alpha-lipoic acid, an antioxidant which helps many diabetics, and is particularly useful for preventing the complication of diabetic neuropathy (damage to nerves from the high blood sugar).[143,144] And I gave him B vitamins, which help regulate blood sugar metabolism. His Vitamin D level was ok, as he was already taking it when he came to see me.

I discussed with Rajiv the possibility of his working more from home, so he could be in control of his food intake for more of the time. As a mere medic, I don't understand the world of international business, and it was a mystery to me why, in the age of Skype and Zoom and all those magic tele-conferencing technologies, he couldn't sit in his house in Paris and conduct meetings from there. But no, he said, I have to go and be there in person.

For a year, the basic treatments outlined above held Rajiv's blood sugar levels where they were, in the low diabetic range while travelling (he tested himself all the time) and even back down to the pre-diabetic range when he was at home. But then the levels he was getting while travelling began to rise, and he got alarmed. He came back to see me, this time with his wife.

I didn't raise the possibility of his eating some eggs or fish or meat, although I think it would have helped immensely – I know when I'm beaten – but I did raise another taboo subject: downsizing. Rajiv's diabetes was only going to get worse if he kept flying round the world, endlessly jet-lagged and unable to control his meals. Diabetes getting worse means damage to the eyes, the heart, the blood vessels and the kidneys. It means skin infections. And it means premature death. Was there any way he could reverse his working pattern, and be at home 75 per cent of the time, and away 25 per cent?

Yes, said his wife, he could. It turned out she'd been asking him to do this for some years. It would mean a massive drop in income, but it would not mean poverty. To my surprise and relief, he agreed almost at once. They exchanged their large house in Paris for a much smaller one, and Rajiv cut his travelling hours back substantially. He was able to stick to his diet and supplement plan most of the time now, and within a year his blood sugar readings were consistently back down into the pre-diabetic range. I am hoping to get them down still further, and am very happy that he chose to prioritise health over wealth. Lastly, I drew Rajiv's attention to the possible links between diabetes and environmental pollution,[145] so he could consider adopting some of the detoxification methods outlined in Chapter 7.

The difference between type 2 diabetes and type 1

In type 2, which Rajiv had, many years of excess sugar consumption, and possibly stress and other factors, cause the body's cells to become "resistant" to insulin. The person's pancreas is still making insulin, the hormone whose job is to send sugar out of the bloodstream and into the cells for use in energy production. But the cells are not "listening" to the insulin any more; they have gone "numb" from experiencing such high insulin levels for so many years (in direct response to excess sugar consumption). So they stop reacting as they should, and don't take sugar in from the bloodstream. So the level of sugar in the blood becomes too high, leading eventually to all the damaging effects listed above. And the cells run short of energy, hence the tiredness so characteristic of diabetes even at the early stages.

This used to be called "mature onset diabetes", but it's happening to younger and younger people, and has become so common that we can rightly call it an epidemic. It's one of the classic diseases of our times, unknown before industrialisation, and entirely preventable.

Type 1 diabetes, or juvenile diabetes, has a different cause. In type 1, the pancreas actually stops making insulin. We think this is because the body's immune system is attacking the cells of the "Islets of Langerhans" within the pancreas, which produce insulin. So it's an autoimmune condition.

Case History: Andrew's Panic Attacks

Andrew was 45, happily married, with a child, and doing a job he enjoyed, when he began experiencing panic attacks "out of nowhere". They could happen anywhere; in the supermarket, on the train to work, even in the garden at home. Day or night. He had seen a psychotherapist but it hadn't helped. "She was really nice, but we couldn't find anything that I was seriously unhappy or anxious about!"

Then he had tried cognitive behaviour therapy, CBT. It had certainly helped him to manage the overwhelming anxiety that gripped him on these occasions, anxiety that seemed to have no content, to not be about anything. The CBT psychologist had taught Andrew some breathing techniques and some "self-talk" techniques that helped him calm down somewhat through these episodes, and to sense when a panic attack was about to happen so he could immediately put the breathing techniques in place. But it had not made the panic attacks any less frequent. It had not solved the problem.

So Andrew came to see me, as a "last resort" and because, he said, "it actually doesn't feel psychological. It feels biological".

In all other respects Andrew seemed well, and there was nothing of note in his past medical history. Then he showed me his one-week food diary. Every day except Sunday, breakfast was a cup of coffee. Every day except Saturday and Sunday, lunch was also a cup of coffee. Most days he had a piece of cake, chocolate bar, doughnut or croissant around 3.00pm. With a coffee. Then dinner in the evening, which was fine.

"But it works for me", he said. "I just don't really get hungry till mid-afternoon."

He wasn't feeling hunger, but I thought he was probably going hypoglycaemic, i.e. his blood sugar was falling too low. Almost the mirror image of Rajiv's problem. When the blood sugar falls too low, as can happen to some people if they haven't eaten all day, the feeling produced can be one of panic, as in Andrew's case; not surprisingly really, because the body thinks you are about to die of starvation. Other people become terribly irritable or even violently angry when their blood sugar drops. It is not so much how **low** it falls that determines these symptoms, but how **fast** it falls. We are not talking here about blood sugar levels so low as to be actually dangerous (as can happen in a type 1 diabetic who has injected their insulin without eating enough food), but in some people the body experiences it as a danger signal – hence the content-free, apparently inexplicable panic attacks.

Well, this was my hypothesis, and now we had to test it. I asked Andrew if he would be prepared to try eating three meals a day for a couple of weeks, and see if the panic attacks went away. He said he was fine with that in principle, but that he was one of those people who just couldn't eat breakfast. He would throw up if he tried to eat anything solid before 11.00am. So we reached a compromise whereby he would take a packed breakfast to work and eat it at 11.00am. Then he would have a late lunch at 3.00pm; a proper meal, instead of his usual sugar hit. And dinner as per usual.

At our second consultation, five weeks later, Andrew reported that his panic attacks were not gone, but were down from about three per week to one a week. His test results told me what it was that remained to be fixed. He was very low in all four of the minerals which help to keep blood sugar stable, namely the trace minerals chromium and manganese, and zinc and magnesium (yes, again!). Also in three of the B vitamins, similarly important for blood sugar regulation. These nutrients were probably low because of Andrew's strange eating (or rather non-eating) patterns. But once depleted by the constant demands of trying to maintain blood sugar levels in a body that isn't being fed, their low levels in turn would make it even harder to keep blood sugar levels stable, and so on, in a vicious circle.

So I gave Andrew supplements of these missing nutrients, all in liquid form except the magnesium and the B complex, and saw him again three months later. His panic attacks had tailed off gradually, and in the past month he had had none at all. Within another three months he could stop all the supplements, as he had normalised his levels and could now maintain them by eating, as he was now doing, three meals a day.

Andrew's case is unusually simple – most patients I see are not nearly so straightforward – but there is a lot to be learnt from it.

Firstly, what I call the "backlog" effect: the hypoglycaemic episodes were not necessarily straight after missing a meal, they could be many hours later. To understand this, we need to know that the pancreas actually produces two hormones to balance our blood sugar: insulin, which lowers the blood sugar level when it goes too high, and glucagon, which raises the blood sugar level when it falls too low. They should work in tandem, a great example of homeostasis.

By hardly eating all day, Andrew was relying heavily on his glucagon just to keep his blood sugar level normal. At some point he would have used up his day's supply of glucagon; the pancreas's capacity to produce it is not infinite. At that point, his insulin would be unopposed – nothing to balance it – and his blood sugar level would crash.

Some people can go without food for much longer than others; everybody's pancreas is different. But Andrew was making things worse by the fact that when he did finally eat, at around 3.00pm, he ate sugar. That sends the blood sugar level straight up, which triggers insulin release, which sends the blood sugar level crashing down, which calls for more production of poor old overworked glucagon. And so on.

The tendency to hypoglycaemia is a recognised medical condition in some European countries, but not in the UK, for some reason. And ditto with low blood pressure. Both conditions are commoner in women than in men. In women, hypoglycaemia occurs quite frequently in the pre-menstrual phase of the cycle, and contributes to irritability, tearfulness and often intense cravings for chocolate. The key thing here is to eat really frequently in the week or so before a period – not sugar, but proper food – to avoid the blood sugar drops that lead to these symptoms, which are real and distressing, although not as dramatic as Andrew's full-blown panic attacks. (In the week leading up to a period, the body doesn't know if you're pregnant or not, so it requires you to eat as though you were, just in case. Go with this need – if you try to resist you'll just end up bingeing on chocolate.)

What about caffeine?

The eagle-eyed among you may have spotted that I did not stop Andrew drinking coffee, which is perhaps surprising. Let me explain. In some people, excess coffee can indeed contribute to panic attacks, and I'll explain how in a minute. But in Andrew's case, I suspected that the problem was not with coffee per se, but with the fact that he was using it as a substitute for food. When he started eating properly, and we normalised the relevant nutrients, his panic attacks, which were really hypoglycaemic episodes, went away, even though he continued to have a coffee with each meal. So there was no need to take away what was for him one of life's pleasures. If proper eating and temporary supplementation had not done the job, then we would indeed have had to look at Andrew withdrawing from caffeine.

These days there are all sorts of clever genetic tests, and we could have used one of them to find out how good Andrew's liver was at detoxifying caffeine. But it is rarely needed, when one can find out by the "Suck it and See" or "Stop it and See" approach. There are indeed people for whom caffeine creates problems; those who are not well able to break it down (detoxify it) in the liver. It can cause migraines, it can keep people up all night. And here's how it can, in some people, contribute to panic attacks.

Caffeine causes adrenalin release in the body. That's why it perks you up and powers you through the day. But too much adrenalin can lead you from useful alertness through mild anxiety to full-blown palpitating, heart-thumping, pouring-with-sweat panic. Not nice. This is the "fight flight fright" mechanism in extremis, a biological state which nature requires only for life-threatening emergencies. Now, whether caffeine does this to you or not depends not only on how much of it you drink, or on how quickly your liver can break it down, but crucially on how quickly your liver can break down adrenalin.

Some people can break down their adrenalin fast; they are usually the calm, placid types. Others can only detox adrenalin very slowly; they are the sort who get stressed easily, and in whom traumatic experiences can result in PTSD, because the stress hormones (adrenalin and noradrenaline) just hang around for ages, un-detoxified.

Just to complicate matters further, adrenalin raises blood sugar levels – because the body thinks it's an emergency. And as we know, when blood sugar shoots up, it then comes crashing back down again, as a result of the action of insulin – and there we go again, with hypoglycaemia. So it looks like panic can actually lead to hypoglycaemia, as well as vice versa, in a vicious circle. And in many people, caffeine isn't necessary for any of this to happen. Their own anxiety or trauma can generate enough adrenalin all on its own.

What about decaffeinated coffee? I wouldn't bother. There are other substances still in decaf coffee which cause similar, adrenalin-inducing effects, and artificial chemicals are used in the decaffeinating process. If you've read all the above, you can probably work out whether coffee is ok for you or not. But if you do drink it, please make sure it's organic and fairly traded.

A final word about panic attacks and psychological therapy for them. For many people, CBT is actually the right approach and very helpful. But it could be even more useful if CBT therapists were more aware of the hypoglycaemia factor, and asked more questions about what their patients are eating (or not eating) and drinking. Andrew was unusual; lots of people who live on coffee and sugar and don't eat proper meals have major social and psychological problems, and they need help with those as well as the dietary changes. Indeed, they may need social/psychological help in order to make the dietary changes possible at all.

Age 50–105: Don't Dement – Prevent! Menopause, Man-O-Pause, Preserving Bone And Brain

Looking after your body has to become a priority now; you can't take its workings for granted any more, but you can certainly help them along. The four golden rules of eating on page 22 apply more than ever now. And here are a couple of tips about drinking – I don't mean alcohol.

Thirst

Thirst signals seem to decrease with age. We don't know why, but the hypothalamus, a small area of the brain which controls thirst (as well as hunger, temperature, hormones, some powerful emotions and the autonomic nervous system) starts forgetting to tell us when we're thirsty. You won't notice this at 50, but you will at 80 – or your children will.

"Mum, this water jug is as full as it was eight hours ago!" is a commonly heard cry.

"But I wasn't thirsty," is the usual reply.

The older we get, the more we need to remind ourselves to keep hydrated. Drink water – preferably filtered. Just Do It. Otherwise we get into a vicious circle; when we dehydrate, our brains dehydrate, so they don't work properly and the thirst signals – and other brain messages – get even fainter.

Sometimes the thirst signals are still there, but they are experienced/interpreted as hunger or sugar cravings rather than thirst. This can happen at any age, but it seems to be commoner in the latter half of life. (The thirst and hunger centres are right next to each other in the hypothalamus.) So people will reach for a snack or a piece of fruit instead of a glass of water. Fruit, of course, provides some water as well as a bit of a sugar hit. (See pages 124–128 for more on the pros and cons of fruit.) If you or your mum or dad seem to be becoming a bit of a fruit-a-holic, it could just be that you/she/he need(s) to be drinking more water, more frequently.

There is something that helps a lot with this; vegetable juicing. It is described in Chapter 7 as part of detoxification, but it has many other uses too, including regulation of thirst sensation, and helping to shift our taste buds "from sweet to green". Many older people who have taken up the practice of making themselves a pint of veg juice in the morning describe how they can now distinguish more clearly between thirst and hunger, and how their craving for sweet things, including fruit juice and fruit, has disappeared. They also say that it keeps them feeling young and healthy, energetic and clear-headed. So it's well worth the effort.

Gums

Becoming "long in the tooth" refers to receding gums and perio-
dontitis or infective gum disease. It is very common but I don't
believe it's inevitable. And it's important to fight it hard, not only
to preserve your teeth and the health of your mouth, but also
because gum disease has been linked to heart disease.[146]

Of course, the basics are important – brushing and flossing after
every meal. Another reason not to snack between meals! But
beyond that? Most dentists recommend mouthwashes and frequent
visits to the hygienist. Have you ever read the ingredients list on
the kind of mouthwash you'd buy in the chemist or supermarket?
It is horrifying. And don't imagine that you're not swallowing
some of it; you are. And anyway, the chemicals in it will get
absorbed into your body via the mucous membranes lining your
mouth. Fortunately, there are safer alternatives. There is an excellent herbal mouthwash from the USA called Periobrite. It works,
but it's expensive; you could instead ask a qualified herbalist
(member of the NIMH) to tell you how to make up one for yourself, from the appropriate herbs. There are many antibacterial
herbs that have been used safely and effectively for centuries, and
you can rinse with those without worrying about what it's doing
to your body.

Additionally, there are three nutrients that are very important
for preserving the health of your gums:

- **Vitamin C** – again! You can take it in the usual way, and also
  rinse with water in which you have dissolved half a teaspoon
  of Vitamin C powder (in the form of magnesium ascorbate –
  details in Chapter 6).

- **Co-Q10**, or Coenzyme Q 10 to give it its full name. It is important for energy production in the mitochondria of all our cells, and especially for the health of our heart and brain (probably because heart and brain cells have so many mitochondria), and for maintaining the integrity of our gums. It's an antioxidant too. So it's the best anti-ageing nutrient around. It occurs naturally in many foods and we can make it in our cells too, but it seems not in sufficient amounts to save our gums or keep our energy levels maximal.

- **L-Lysine**. An amino acid, so it occurs in protein foods, but again not in sufficient quantities to treat sore gums. Lysine helps with cold sores and mouth ulcers as well.

Oil-pulling for gum health

You have to be really dedicated to your gums to do this one. Melt some coconut oil (doesn't take long; it melts on a hot summer's day) and rinse with it. Rinse, spit and change the oil, rinse, spit and so on, for 10 minutes. But don't spit the oil into the wash-basin – it will solidify and block the drains! Spit it into a tissue and put it in the bin. I have some patients who are devoted to this practice and have been doing it for years, for 10 or even 20 minutes a night, and swear it's what's keeping their gums in tip-top condition. They do it before bed while listening to the radio. I have other patients who say life's too short to spend 10 minutes a day doing stuff like this. Growing old is partly about finding the balance between doing things that improve your health, and thus increase the quality and

> length of your life, and actually living your life. It's a very
> individual choice. I think part of the knack is learning to enjoy
> things like veg juicing and mouth rinsing; doing them
> consciously and mindfully rather than in a rush and resentfully.
> Easier once you've retired, of course.

Two final tips about preserving your gums (and thus your teeth):

- Tea-tree oil, an "essential oil" you can buy in any good health-food shop, is a very powerful antibacterial, antifungal and antiviral. It's totally natural but it does smell like hospital antiseptic, and it's too strong to use neat. But you can put a drop or two in your mouthwash, whether that's a herbal one or the coconut oil, and it adds greatly to keeping your mouth free of unfriendly bugs.

- You can now get "mouth probiotics", good bacteria of the kind that are supposed to live in a healthy mouth. Remember, the mouth is part of the gut; it's the beginning of the digestive tract. So the same principles apply that we've discussed in relation to the gut as a whole: good bugs in, bad bugs out, and no sugar!

Exercise

I'm not going to go into much detail about exercise, because there are dozens of good books about it, and an excellent section in Dr Rangan Chatterjee's *The 4 Pillar Plan*. Just five short things to say:

1 Keep moving! You can't be healthy in body or mind if you don't move.

2 Please be sensible. If you are 70 and have never done any exercise before, don't start off with a 5-mile jog. Build up to it gradually.

3 You don't need to join a gym. The best place to exercise is in the park. It's free and there's more oxygen. Just walk. Or run or cycle. Or do Yoga or Tai Chi. Or dance or Pilates. Or all of the above. Or go swimming.

4 At the time of writing, there is a fashion for High-Intensity Interval Training (HIIT), short bursts of very intensive aerobic exercise. It suits some people but not others. If you're doing it already, that's fine. If not, and if you're over 65, I would give it a miss.

5 Specifically for prevention of osteoporosis, about which more below, exercise needs to be weight-bearing. If you are thin you can do your exercise wearing a backpack, and gradually increase the amount of weight you put in it. If you are fat, all exercise is already weight-bearing exercise! But hopefully, as you exercise and cut out sugar and refined carbs, you'll lose the weight, and then you'll need the backpack.

Sunlight

Exposure to sunlight is essential at every age,[147] but the housebound elderly are particularly at risk of sunlight deprivation. If you or someone you love are stuck at home unable to get out, please get the GP to check your Vitamin D levels once or twice a year, and take a Vitamin D supplement accordingly.

Menopause

Some women sail through and hardly notice anything except that their periods have stopped. Others suffer terribly with hot flushes, vaginal dryness, weight gain, anxiety, depression, memory loss – the full works. Most are somewhere in between. There is also the worry that with the drop in levels of the female hormones (oestrogen and progesterone) the bones may start to thin – osteoporosis.

The hypothalamus, which I mentioned earlier in connection with the sensation of thirst, is also in charge here. Or rather, not so much in charge as in chaos. As the ovaries stop producing oestrogen and progesterone, the pituitary gland (just below the hypothalamus in the brain) responds by producing vast amounts of FSH (follicle stimulating hormone) and LH (luteinising hormone), in a futile attempt to get the ovaries' hormone production started again. During the menstruating years, there is a negative feedback cycle between the ovaries and the pituitary, and that's what winds down at the menopause. The very high levels of FSH and LH are what is measured in a blood test to confirm "menopausal status", although in most situations the test is not needed.

But the pituitary in turn receives its hormonal instructions from the hypothalamus directly above it. The very high levels of FSH and LH feed back to the hypothalamus too, and it behaves very temperamentally; remember the hypothalamus controls temperature (hence hot flushes), thirst, hunger and powerful emotions.

All of which can go awry at the menopause. So, just as adolescents can justifiably say, "It's not me, it's my brain!", a woman going through the menopause can truthfully say, "It's my hypothalamus that's in meltdown!"

I suspect that oestrogen and progesterone are not the only hormones which decline at menopause. They may decline the most dramatically, but other hormones such as growth hormone and thyroid hormone, both also controlled ultimately by the hypothalamus, may gradually decrease too, and in men as well as in women.

So here's what I do when women come to me with these very distressing menopausal symptoms. It's potentially a 5-stage process, although most people will only need stages 1, 2 and maybe 3. It's based on the principles already enunciated in this book, especially in the Introduction, because the menopause is experienced as a far more disabling and "ill-making" phenomenon when a woman's nutrition is already poor, than when it is tip-top.

Stage 1: Apply the four golden rules (see page 22). Then check the gut. Is the bowel working perfectly? Is she absorbing all her minerals and vitamins properly? Are there unfriendly gut bugs in there, producing waste products that make the "brain fog" so much worse? So everything said in Chapter 2 about TTCs applies here.

Stage 2: I would consider the nutrients that are most essential at this life stage. They are:

- **Vitamin E** – almost always low in women struggling with the menopause, and giving it as a supplement for a few months really helps.

- **EFAs (essential fatty acids)**, both omega 3 and omega 6, especially evening primrose oil, which is an omega 6.

- **All the B vitamins**, especially B12.

- **Vitamin D, Vitamin K2 and all the minerals – zinc and magnesium especially** – for preventions of osteoporosis.

For women who don't want or can't afford blood tests, I would simply recommend taking all of these nutrients anyway.

All the above makes a significant difference to at least 50 per cent of women. For the other 50 per cent, whom it helps but not enough, I would proceed as follows:

Stage 3: Enquiring about toxins. This might very occasionally entail blood tests, but usually it just means taking a detailed chemical/environmental/occupational history, asking really awkward questions like:

- Do you dye your hair?

- Do you use perfume?

- Do you use deodorant?

- Have you ever worked in a factory or laboratory?

- Have you ever had to spray your house/flat for mice, ants or wasp nests?

🌿 Have you used weed-killer in the garden?

🌿 Do you use powerful oven-cleaners?

🌿 Have you got metal amalgam fillings in your teeth?

And dozens more. Of course, toxic chemicals getting into us, through the skin or through inhalation, is damaging at any life-stage, and most damaging pre-natally and in infancy, but for some reason they do also seem to cause a lot of problems around the time of menopause. So it's a good moment for a review.

Women are shocked to hear that their favourite hair dye, perfume or deodorant is full of dangerous chemicals. I was shocked too when I first began to realise. Just take your magnifying glass, read the list of ingredients and look them up. Hair dyes go straight through the scalp into the bloodstream, and have been linked to bladder cancer and breast cancer (see references 156, 157 and 236). Perfumes contain benzene and other potentially carcinogenic petrochemicals – straight into your body and brain via the nose, lungs and skin. But you can safely use natural essential oils instead, such as lavender, jasmine, rose, geranium and more.

Deodorants, even without the hormone-mimicking Parabens, are still hazardous. Look very carefully even if it says "aluminium-free". Some so-called "natural" or "herbal" deodorants contain "alum". Even it says "rock crystal alum", it is still aluminium by another name. The armpit is very near the breast, and deposits of aluminium have been found in cancerous breast tumours.[148] And aluminium is also implicated in Alzheimer's disease.[149]

When a woman is prepared to let go of these chemicals, then

it's worth doing a thorough detox programme, as described in Chapter 7, and this, on top of the nutritional work-up, tends to solve the menopausal problems in about another 30 per cent of people. That leaves a "hard core" of about 20 per cent, with whom it is necessary to proceed to stage 4.

Stage 4: At this point I would refer the patient on to a medical herbalist, a member of the NIMH. Having put gut health, nutrition and detoxification in place, a good herbalist will almost always be able to complete the job. After all, herbalists have been helping with "women's problems" since way before we knew anything about the biochemistry of hormones. These days herbalists do in fact know about the biochemistry of hormones, and the biochemistry of plants, too, and can combine their scientific knowledge with centuries of accumulated wisdom and clinical experience.

Stage 5: Very few women, even after all of the above, will still be suffering with menopausal symptoms. These women, and these only, I would refer on for "bio-identical hormone replacement therapy". It is different from conventional HRT in that the hormones used have exactly the same molecular structure as those produced naturally in the human body. The bio-identical oestrogen is made from wild yams, whereas in conventional HRT the oestrogen is extracted from horses' urine. Horses' biology is not the same as ours. The bio-identical progesterone is actually progesterone, whereas conventional HRT mostly uses a progestogen, a synthetic molecule, that doesn't occur naturally in the body.

The NHS is beginning to provide bio-identical HRT in some areas. You'd have to ask. Some women find this treatment transformational, others don't. But what about the risks? There are long-term studies showing the very real dangers of conventional HRT,[150] but it's simply too early to say how much safer the bio-identical version is. One small study showed a lot of benefits and an absence of side effects,[151] but, as the saying goes, more research is needed.

Preserving bone, preventing osteoporosis

Some women's bone does get thinner after the menopause; more porous, less dense. Slight thinning is called osteopenia, and more marked thinning is called osteoporosis. It's not a clinical diagnosis, it's a radiological one. In other words, you don't **feel** any different; it can only be seen on X-ray. But it can lead to major fractures (particularly of hip or wrist) from a minor fall, and can also lead to collapse of the vertebrae, with back pain and loss of height as a result.

One of the things we don't know about osteoporosis is whether to think of it as a pathology or as a change that occurs inevitably with age. It's usually only diagnosed when a person has a fall and therefore an X-ray. We don't know how many older women have been walking around with osteoporosis for decades but have never had a fracture. One patient of mine whom I was treating for osteoporosis said that her mother had had osteoporosis from her 50s into her 90s, and had been perfectly alright. Nevertheless, osteoporotic hip fractures can be disabling and even fatal, so we need to do what we can. Here's what I find helps:

1 First, you've guessed it, **Vitamin D**. In a woman with known osteoporosis, I would aim to keep the blood levels of Vitamin D towards the upper end of the normal range, i.e. between 150 and 200 nmol/l. Vitamin D facilitates the absorption of calcium from the gut into the bloodstream.

2 Second, you need **Vitamin K2**. This helps to transfer calcium from the bloodstream into the bone. So they work together. If you eat your greens, friendly gut bugs will make some Vitamin K2 for you, but it may not be enough.

3 Then you need all the **minerals** that bone needs.[152] But calcium supplements risk depleting magnesium, which bone also needs. If your Vitamin D level is good, you will absorb enough calcium from your food. Bone contains other minerals as well as calcium, and many trace elements such as zinc, copper and boron are needed for its metabolism; bone is a living tissue. There are plenty of combination supplements with all the relevant minerals in, with names like Osteo-Aid, Osteo-Food and so on. As ever, check the ingredients list and avoid added junk.

4 You also need weight-bearing **exercise**, as above.

5 Very importantly, you need a sufficient level of **stomach acid** to absorb all those minerals. But after age 50 our stomach acid production begins to fall, and this may in fact be one of the contributing factors in osteoporosis. So squeeze a lemon or lime onto every main meal, or take a little apple cider vinegar (in warm water, with a little honey if needed); then you'll absorb the minerals from your food and your supplements, and they'll reach your bones. This means that unfortunately, if you are taking acid-suppressing drugs for reflux or similar conditions, you are more at risk of osteoporosis. Steroid drugs also carry this risk.

Then there's the problem of **fluoride**. There is plenty of evidence that fluoride interferes with the architecture of bone.[153] Overall, fluoride appears to increase bone density but it also, oddly, increases the rate of bone fractures,[154] which rather defeats the object, and shows us how much we still don't know about the mechanisms of osteoporotic fractures. There's fluoride in your toothpaste, unless you're careful to buy a fluoride-free version – see page 166. Depending where you live, there may also be fluoride added to your tap water. It is added to tap water in most parts of the USA, but in very few countries in Europe. More on this in Chapter 7. If you've been unwittingly consuming fluoride for a while, you can start filtering your tap water now, and taking kelp or iodine will gradually remove the fluoride from your system.

6 Lastly, there is a view that too much animal protein contributes to osteoporosis.[155] So it's probably a good idea to go easy on the meat. Once or twice a week is plenty for most of us anyway. Organic and free-range, of course.

Once I've put all these measures in place, I ask the patient to repeat their bone density scan in two years' time. Usually we find that the bone density has held stable. Then we keep calm and carry on with the regime, and repeat the bone scan after a further three years. One doesn't want to do it too often; it is radiation, after all. Sometimes it's still holding stable, other times it's actually improved, which is fantastic. In only one case have I found that it continued to decline, and that was in someone who had had a very early menopause, aged 38. I referred her for bio-identical hormone therapy and we found that the hormones, combined with continuing the supplement and exercise regime, held her bone density stable and then eventually improved it.

Man-o-pause

Sorry guys, I don't think this really exists. There is no male event equivalent to the menopause. Men just age gradually and steadily, but they have to work just as hard as women do to remain fit and healthy. They can occasionally get osteoporosis too, and the same treatment approach would apply. And doctors who work with bio-identical hormones can use testosterone too, if appropriate.

The real purpose of this section is to explain how, if you have a female partner, you can support her through the menopause. It's simple. Remember, hair dyes are toxic.[156,157] So are perfumes and almost all deodorants. So is nail varnish, if she puts it on indoors and inhales the fumes. Ditto nail varnish remover. Most make-up is toxic too – check the ingredients list! – and foundation stops the sun from reaching the skin of the face and making Vitamin D. Hair spray – very nasty. And so on. Your role, ideally, is to convince her that she doesn't need all that stuff. That you will love her just as much with white hair and real skin and real nails, and the real smell of a human being. We can re-acclimatise to the smell of human sweat. Not old, smelly sweat – we can wash every day – but fresh sweat. It never hurt anyone, and it's our natural method of detoxing. Whereas the chemicals we use to stop ourselves from sweating are not safe at all.

So figure out how much money can be saved by letting go of all those forms of disguise; maybe you can have an extra holiday together. Tell her that you love her just the way she is; and stick around. Be there. Tell her also that you'd rather have her fit and healthy than trying to conform to some advertiser's ideal of false youth and beauty. And, paradoxically, unless she mentions it first, Don't Mention the Menopause!

And while you're at it, ditch the aftershave.

Preserving brain, preventing dementia

The brain is part of the body, and to stay healthy it needs good nutrition, a clean, non-toxic environment and plenty of exercise. When I say exercise, I mean both mental and physical. Yes, you need to stay mentally active – "use it or lose it" – but that's not enough; the brain needs you to be physically active too.

At time of writing, 850,000 people in the UK have the diagnosis of Alzheimer's disease or some other form of dementia. And many more probably have the disease without yet having the diagnosis. That's close to a million people. It is a tragedy, a disaster and a scandal. While researchers are busily engaged in the futile but lucrative search for a cure, I think it's urgent to focus on causes and prevention.[158,159]

But first, we need to examine what we are usually told about it. "It's because we have an ageing population," goes the story. "We are living longer, so we are living long enough to get these diseases of ageing."

There are several reasons why this explanation is wrong. Firstly, we are not actually living longer than our mid-19th-century Victorian ancestors did. They ate better than we think and lived to a greater age than we think.[160] The myth arose because of the way mortality rates are calculated. The **average** age of death in Victorian times was indeed much younger than it is now, but that's because the **average figure included child mortality**. A very high proportion of children died from infectious diseases under the age of five, and their deaths brought the **average** age of death right down to the 40s. It's just arithmetic. So it looks at first glance as though very few people survived into their 80s and 90s. But in fact plenty of them did, and they mostly kept their marbles.[161,162]

Secondly, the disease that Alzheimer described he actually called "**pre**-senile dementia"; the patient in whom he first observed it was 51. In other words, it was about people suffering cognitive decline at a much younger age than you would expect. If someone starts struggling to recall their acquaintances' names at the age of 93, we don't worry too much. But at 53 it's a cause for grave concern. And this is what we're seeing; cognitive decline in middle age, not just in old age.

Thirdly, there is a logical contradiction in an argument that says, essentially, "Thanks to the wonders of modern medicine, we are now living long enough to get terribly ill."

Dementia on the scale we are seeing now is unprecedented. When a disease increases in frequency so rapidly in one or two generations, it means that genetics are playing only a tiny part in it. Most people with dementia today did not have a parent with dementia. It means that environmental and nutritional factors, i.e. changes in the way we are living, must be playing the major part.

As a modern epidemic, its causes are similar to those of diabetes (indeed, dementia has been called "diabetes type 3" or "diabetes of the brain"), heart disease, cancer and so on. But the brain has particular vulnerabilities, which help us to pinpoint some specific causative factors.

The brain contains lots of fat. All its nerve cells are surrounded and protected by fat. So it has a particular need for good fats, of the kinds found in oily fish, avocado, nuts, seeds, egg yolk, coconut oil, hempseed oil and so on. The fashion for low-fat diets over the past 40–50 years has a lot to answer for. In the attempt to lose weight, people starved their brain of the good fat molecules it needed. And when they did eat fat, it was toxic fat: the hydrogen ated vegetable oils in margarine and so many processed foods, and the dangerous trans fats produced by cooking with vegetable oils at high temperatures. Ironically, chips fried in lard were safer than chips fried in vegetable oil.

Furthermore, people replaced those fats with sugar, hence "diabetes of the brain".

Another consequence of the brain being composed largely of fats is that lipophilic toxins, i.e. those which dissolve in fat, will find their way into the brain. These fat-soluble poisons include many petrochemicals like benzene, and are found in everything from car fumes to cosmetics. They are even in the standard mois-turising creams people put on babies with eczema – and they go right in; through the skin, through the bloodstream, through the blood-brain barrier.

Two heavy metals in particular seem to gravitate towards the brain and to be implicated in dementia: mercury and aluminium. Others pose risks as well, including cadmium (from cigarette smoke mostly) and nickel. Recent studies link air pollution with dementia (see Chapter 7), and we will see more such studies. That's the tiny molecule nitrogen dioxide, as well as the fat-soluble chemicals described above, doing the damage.

And then there are the missing nutrients. The most important ones for preventing brain decline are: all the B vitamins, especially B12 and, yet again, the sunshine vitamin, Vitamin D. Significantly, Vitamin D is a fat-soluble vitamin, as are vitamins A, E and K. Any diet low in fats will make it very unlikely that the body is absorbing enough of these vitamins, so the poor old brain will be starved of them.

Now finally, and rather more cheerfully, let's look at a case history where some of this knowledge was put into practice, with a positive outcome.

Case History: Sylvie's Dementia

Sylvie was a lawyer from West Africa, who had been living and working in the north-west of England for over 30 years. She was 54 when she came to see me, anxious and tearful, having noticed that she was forgetting nouns, losing concentration, struggling to spell words she'd been able to spell easily all her life, and occasionally getting lost in the middle of a sentence she was saying. On one occasion, she had turned up at court at the wrong time, and on another with the wrong client's papers.

The brighter people are, the sooner they notice the signs of their own cognitive decline. It was still subtle, and Sylvie was well able to bluff and cover up. Her colleagues hadn't noticed anything, and she hadn't been to her GP; but she knew. Usually there are several causative factors combining to create this degree of memory loss, and that is what I found.

Firstly, I found the lowest level of Vitamin D I had ever seen. Remember, the normal range is 75–200 nmol/l. Sylvie's level was not 60 or 40 or 25. It was 5. Almost not there. I ordered a repeat of the test, to be certain (the lab repeated it free of charge because they too were astounded and understood its significance) and it came back the same: 5.0.

How had it got to be so drastically low? For four reasons:

1 The north-west of England has a high level of cloud cover. Its relative lack of sunlight has been linked to an increased prevalence of heart disease,[163] but the low levels of Vitamin D that result from lack of sunlight have implications for many other diseases as well. And there was no sunshine inside the courtroom either.

2 Combining crucially with the lack of sunshine, Sylvie was very dark-skinned. She needed **more** sunshine than a lighter-skinned person, in order to manufacture enough Vitamin D.

3 Although Sylvie wasn't a vegan or even a vegetarian, she disliked fish intensely and never ate it, so she lost an important food source of Vitamin D.

4 She had been dieting on and off for 25 years, always trying low-fat diets. So she'd missed out on Vitamin D in that way too, as well as missing out on the good fats themselves.

This low level of Vitamin D was serious enough; no one could have normal cognitive function with such a low level, and I had no way of knowing how long it had been so low – probably for decades. But I found another factor as well. Sylvie had a very high level of aluminium in her urine, and aluminium also showed up in a "Melisa" test for heavy metals. Aluminium is a known neurotoxin. When it accumulates in us slowly over many years, we call it chronic toxicity, and it is a known causative factor in Alzheimer's disease.[164,165] More well-known, perhaps, is the episode of acute aluminium toxicity that occurred at Camelford in Cornwall in 1988; aluminium sulphate got into the town's water supply, and the authorities took 16 days to inform the residents about the contamination. Numerous local people were affected by serious neurological and psychiatric symptoms, many of which continue to this day, and there was at least one death.

Aluminium belongs in the crust of the earth, not inside us. How had so much aluminium got into Sylvie's body? On careful questioning we found four possible sources:

⚑ First, she cooked in aluminium saucepans. Not only that, but she made a lot of tomato sauce, which is acidic, and therefore would leach out some of the aluminium. And she kept it in the pan for a day or two, plenty of time for the aluminium to leak into the food.

* Secondly, Sylvie used a lot of underarm deodorant. "It's hot in court," she said. She showed me the roll-on canister. Yes, it contained aluminium, as well as several other nasties.

* Thirdly, Sylvie kept leftovers in the fridge wrapped in aluminium foil. She took lunch to work wrapped in aluminium foil and she cooked her Sunday roast – with lemon squeezed on it – wrapped in aluminium foil. Lemon juice is acid and would leach the aluminium out into the food.

* Fourthly, a source Sylvie herself pointed out, once we got talking about aluminium. Sylvie had had the Hepatitis B jab and a few other vaccinations – she couldn't remember which – for travelling to visit family in Africa. She didn't feel too good straight after the jabs, and being a lawyer, she'd asked the nurse if she could look at the manufacturer's insert in the vaccine pack. She looked at it, but not being a chemist she couldn't remember the names of all the additives that were in there along with the virus. But she did remember seeing aluminium.

It is thought that we only absorb a small proportion of any aluminium that we swallow. But aluminium in a vaccine (it is used as an "adjuvant" to stimulate the immune response) is going straight into the body – and the brain.

Sylvie had three other contributing factors. Her long-term low-fat diet had deprived the brain of good fats, and her excessive sugar consumption had done the brain no good either (and it had also stopped her losing weight). Finally, there was the air pollution factor; she spent a lot of her time in central Liverpool and central Manchester. But that was one thing I couldn't change. I was just deeply grateful that she didn't have any metal amalgam fillings in her teeth, so at least we weren't dealing with mercury toxicity as well.

I gave Sylvie Vitamin D3, lots of it, over a long period. I gave her the full 7-part detox protocol described in Chapter 7, to get rid of the aluminium, along with lots of Vitamin C for the same purpose. I also gave her a very specific supplement that is excellent at pulling aluminium out of the body: natural silica. Silica has a chemical affinity with aluminium; it bonds with it and removes it. I gave Sylvie silica as a nutritional supplement, but there are two other ways of doing it too. First, the herbal remedy horsetail contains a lot of silica, so that works too. Second, certain mineral waters are naturally high in silica, so they can help as well.

I pleaded with Sylvie to start eating some good-fat foods, although it went very much against the grain for her after years of having been indoctrinated with the low-fat fashion. But she did it, and she also cut out sugar.

Lastly, I gave her a B complex, B12, magnesium, zinc, phosphatidyl choline, and some fish oil capsules alternating with evening primrose oil capsules. The reason for alternating them is that fish oils (omega 3 essential fatty acids) and evening primrose oil (omega 6 essential fatty acids) are both processed by the body into natural anti-inflammatory substances. The first step of this process is carried out by an enzyme called delta-6-desaturase. But the enzyme can't work on them both at once. The brain needs both omega 3 and omega 6 EFAs, but you get more mileage out of taking them separately, e.g. one at breakfast and the other at dinner. Sylvie particularly urgently needed the fish oil, as she didn't eat any fish at all.

Sylvie was the perfect patient, and she stuck with her admittedly complex and demanding regime to the letter. She also decided to see a neurologist, who did extensive verbal testing and a CT scan of the brain. He gave her a diagnosis of early-stage Alzheimer's. She held her nerve. A year later, we retested her nutrient and toxin levels. The Vitamin D and other nutrients had normalised, and the aluminium was gone. Her mood was much better, and her memory problems were unchanged. "Unchanged" may not sound like much, but the normal pattern would have been progressive deterioration. We had prevented that, thus far. It is extremely difficult to reverse brain damage, but it is often possible to prevent further damage occurring.

Another year on, Sylvie went back to the neurologist. On inter-viewing her again he found no change, but to his surprise and puzzlement the brain scan actually showed a tiny improvement; some of the tell-tale white patches were gone. Sylvie's incipient Alzheimer's disease was caught at a relatively early stage. This is crucial. Just as prevention is better than cure, so attempting treat-ment at an early stage is far more likely to be successful than if it's left till later.

Many years on, Sylvie is managing fine at work and feeling happy. There has still been no deterioration. Given her desperately low initial level of Vitamin D, I decided to send her for a bone scan to check for osteoporosis. It did indeed show osteoporosis, and we are managing that too, as described above. Sylvie does a lot of physical exercise now, both before and after work, to preserve her brain and her bones. As a bonus, she's finally lost the weight she never managed to lose in all the years of that destructive low-fat diet.

CHAPTER 6
NOURISH AND
FLOURISH

Safe and Sensible Supplementing of Nutrients

First of all, do we actually need nutritional supplements? The short answer is: some of us do, some of the time. But why? Why can't we get all the nourishment we need from food?

Here's why: the soil in which our food is grown has been depleted of nutrients by decades of intensive farming with fertilisers and pesticides. Then our food is transported, stored and wrapped in plastic. And many of us are not digesting or absorbing it well. And the amount of nutrients our bodies require has been greatly increased by stress, pollution and numerous other aspects of 21st century life. So the gap between what we need and what's in our food is growing wider.

Of course, supplements can never be a **substitute** for good food, fresh air, exercise, sufficient sleep and so on. But they may be a necessary **add-on** to those things, at certain moments in our lives. So this chapter will tell you how to choose them, what to look for, what to avoid. When to take them, which to combine, which not to combine. It will also discuss the pros and cons of multi-vits and multi-minerals, and the government's recommended daily allowances of vitamins and minerals.

When choosing supplements, you are looking for maximum nutrients with minimum rubbish – and this is a challenge. By "rubbish" I mean the astonishing amounts of fillers, flavours, colours, coatings, binding agents, lubricants, thickeners, stabilisers, preservatives and anti-caking agents that many cheap supplements contain. Some of these substances are also used in the building and decorating trades, and in cosmetics. Pharmaceutical medicines often contain more and worse ones. You don't want to be swallowing these chemicals along with your vitamins and minerals; it rather defeats the object. They are put in there primarily to make life easier for the purveyors of mass market supplements; they allow the manufacturing process to be totally mechanised – quicker, cheaper, less labour-intensive. And by filling up their capsules/tablets with bulking agents, the manufacturers put more money in their own pockets, and more rubbish and fewer nutrients into your body. So here are some tips to avoid the junk and get a higher proportion of nutrients from your supplements.

Don't go to the supermarket or chemist. Don't even go to the kind of health-food shop that sells only its own brand of supplements. Go to a health-food shop that stocks a wide variety of brands, take your time and TAKE YOUR MAGNIFYING GLASS!

Be very careful when reading the label. You're not just looking under "Nutritional Information" or even where it says "This tablet contains"; those will only tell you about the nutrients, not the junk. You need to read the actual "Ingredients". If the supplement you are looking at comes in a box, remember, a box has six sides; you may need to read all six of them to find the complete ingredients list, and it may be in tiny print. On the bottle of one popular multi-vit marketed at children, I searched in vain for the full ingredients list. Eventually I realised that one had to pull back a tiny, well-hidden flap, and unpeel the label, to reveal a lot of stuff I wouldn't want anybody's kiddies swallowing. Very different from the jolly impression one got from the colourful label on the front of the bottle.

Similarly, if you are ordering online, make sure you can see the full ingredients list; not just what's **in** the capsule, but also what the capsule itself is made of. If you find yourself interested in a particular product, look at the ingredients lists of a few other supplements made by the same company; you'll get a clearer idea of how much they rely on artificial additives. Unfortunately, there's no such thing as a free lunch, and the better quality supplements (more nutrients, less rubbish) will cost more.

Here are some of the additives commonly used in nutritional supplements. Some are harmless, some are not, and on some the jury is still out.

- **Talc**. I kid you not. Yes, it's talcum powder.

- **Stearic acid/magnesium stearate**. It's a saturated fat used as a lubricant. A few people, often those with ME/Chronic Fatigue Syndrome, have allergic reactions to it. But it's one of the hardest to avoid.

- **Titanium dioxide**. A white dye, also used in paint and sunscreen and as a food colouring. Totally unnecessary, and best avoided.

🌿 **Dicalcium phosphate**. This may well turn out to be problematic.[166]

🌿 **Potassium sorbate**. A preservative that can spark off hay fever or asthma in certain sensitive individuals.

🌿 **Ascorbyl palmitate**. Another lubricant.

🌿 **Methyl paraben**. This is a preservative and fungicide which is also, unfortunately, an oestrogen mimic and an anti-androgen.

🌿 **Citric acid**. Don't imagine they get this by squeezing oranges and lemons. They make it from mould.

🌿 **Benzoic acid/benzoate**. Alright for many people in small amounts, but some people do have allergic reactions to it even though it is a naturally occurring substance.

🌿 **Sucralose (Splenda)**. An artificial sweetener made by taking a molecule of ordinary sugar, sucrose, and replacing three of its hydroxyl (hydrogen + oxygen) groups with chlorine atoms. Research shows it may well be problematic,[167,168] and it may be problematic for the planet as a whole, not just for the individuals consuming it. At high temperatures, e.g. in municipal incinerators, it decomposes to produce dioxins and dibenzofurans,[169] which are carcinogens as well as endocrine disruptors, and are among the deadliest chemicals known. Dioxins are the chemicals that were released in the Seveso disaster of 1976; thousands of animals died, several children were taken to hospital, and effects on adults included the skin disease chloracne, and still many years later an increased rate of cancer and diabetes, and also low sperm counts in young men who had been in the womb at the time of the accident.

- **Caramel**. Burnt sugar.

- **Malto-dextrin**. Glucose syrup – a synthetic starch – effectively a form of sugar.

- **"Flavour"**. This could be anything. They're not legally required to tell you.

- **"Natural flavouring"**. As above. "Natural" and "Natural Source" have become virtually meaningless in this context. Everything is ultimately from a natural source, but chemical processing can turn it into a different substance with totally different properties.

- **Guar gum**. A thickening, stabilising powder made from guar beans.

- **Acacia gum**. Gum arabic – probably ok for most people.

- **Iron oxide**. Essentially this is rust. A probably harmless but needless colouring.

🖉 **Silicon dioxide**. This is silica, used as a harmless anti-caking agent.

🖉 **Calcium carbonate**. This is basically limestone, or chalk. Although it's harmless in itself, if it is the first or second ingredient on the list then it's being used as a cheap filler, and you are getting much less in the way of actual vitamins or absorbable minerals.

🖉 **Glycerol/Glycerine**. A sweetener.

But what about the capsule?
There tends to be rather less junk in capsules than in tablets (less need for sticky "binders"), but what is the capsule shell made of? Here there is very little wriggle-room. It tends to be either a vegetable source or gelatine. "Vegetable" capsules are made of one or more of the following three compounds, all synthetic:

🖉 **Microcrystalline cellulose**. Sounds like plant fibre, and essentially it is, but it's more like wood-pulp than a leaf. It seems most people can cope with it ok.

🖉 **Hypromellose**. This is short for Hydroxy-Propyl-Methyl Cellulose or HPMC; also from plant fibre, but problematic for some people.

🖉 **Cross-linked cellulose gum**. This is also known as sodium croscarmellose or sodium Carboxy-Methyl Cellulose (CMC).

Most people's digestive systems can manage these, but it's a question of quantity. Smaller capsules are easier to swallow, of course, and easier on the gut all the way down. And sometimes you can open the capsules and mix the contents with water or food (eg yogurt), but ONLY IF IT SAYS YOU CAN. Responsible manufacturers will tell you on the packaging or the bottle whether it's safe to do this. It often is, but **never** in the case of digestive enzymes or hydrochloric acid supplements that could burn the oesophagus (gullet).

The other material from which capsules can be made is **gelatine**. This is actually a far more natural substance, and easy to digest, but it comes from a pig (or sometimes a cow), so of course it is not acceptable if your diet is vegetarian, vegan, kosher or halal. Occasionally you can find capsules made of fish gelatine, which would be alright for people whose diet is kosher or halal.

The **order** in which the ingredients are listed is important. Whatever's first, there's most of that. If the first two or three ingredients on the list are some version of sugar, or bulking agents like calcium carbonate, or if you see more than two or three of the dodgier items listed above, then save your pennies and put it back on the shelf. The vitamins or minerals or essential fatty acids you are after should be first on the list, not right at the end in tiny amounts, among a load of "E" numbers! On the other hand, if an ingredient constitutes less than 1 per cent of the total contents, then it doesn't have to be declared on the label at all!

Wherever possible, get your supplements in liquid or powder form; then you haven't got the capsule shells to contend with. This isn't possible for all supplements, but where it is, it can be easier on your gut. Liquids are better absorbed anyway, especially minerals like zinc, selenium, chromium and manganese. You can also feed liquid minerals to the sproutlings on your window ledge (see pages 76–77).

With regard to the vitamin and mineral content of supplements, more is more; you want max nutrients and ideally zero junk. But how much is the right amount? What dose of each vitamin/mineral/EFA do you need? Of course it depends on your age, size and health situation, but I'll try to give some general guidance. First, however, we need briefly to examine the UK government's recommendations.

Recommended daily amounts (RDAs)

The government produces RDAs for most nutrients. For vitamins and minerals, these are now called nutrient reference values, or NRVs. But the numbers are the same, and you can easily look them up. They are still based on the outdated science I learnt in medical school, namely that we just need vitamins to prevent deficiency diseases. So the government recommendation is, for example, 1.1 mg of Vitamin B1 (Thiamine) daily. That will indeed prevent you getting Beriberi. But it doesn't take account of the fact that you may be losing the B vitamins hand-over-fist from stress, or from excessive consumption of alcohol or refined carbohydrate. Nor does it take into account the wide spectrum that exists between total health and a full-blown, fatal deficiency disease. And thirdly, it does not – and cannot – take into account the great biochemical variation between individuals, which means that different people have vastly differing requirements for particular vitamins and minerals; genetic testing and clinical experience demonstrate this again and again.

Similarly, the government's recommendation of 2.5 **micro**grams of vitamin B12 daily will prevent most people from getting Pernicious Anaemia, but for some people it is not nearly enough for optimal mental clarity and physical energy. One more example: the government's NRV for Vitamin C is 80 mg a day. This will stop you getting scurvy. But it is not enough to ward off infections or late-life gum disease or cancer, and it ignores the fact that the Vitamin C we take in gets destroyed by tea, coffee, cigarettes, alcohol, paracetamol and stress.

On most supplement pots, you will see what percentage of the government's NRV that supplement gives you. Some supplements will provide, for example, the B vitamins at levels quite close to the government's recommendations, between 1 and 2 mg for most of them. Others will supply 50 or even 100 mg of most of the B vitamins. The lower doses optimistically assume perfect absorption from the gut. The higher doses don't rely on good absorption but they do rely, correctly, on the fact that the B vitamins, like Vitamin C, are water-soluble; you cannot overdose, because you simply pee out what you don't use. So if you see that the amount of B12 in a supplement is 1000 per cent or even 10,000 per cent of the government's NRV, don't panic. It's because the NRV is tiny, not because the supplement is over-the-top.

So in terms of the B vitamins, most people are fine to take the doses found in any good-quality, junk-free B complex, which is usually 50 mg of most members of the B group. Needs for Vitamin C vary hugely; some people are fine with 500 mg twice a day in winter and none in the summer. Others need vastly more, and benefit from it.

With the minerals and the fat-soluble vitamins one has to

exercise more caution, as overdose is theoretically possible. With Vitamin A, the government recommendation of 800 ug (2664 iu) is in fact enough, and we can get it from food, so we don't need it in a supplement. With Vitamin D, the amount you need really should be determined by a blood test result; you want to keep your blood level of Vitamin D between 75 and 200 nmol/l. For most people this means taking about 2000 iu each evening through the winter, but none in the summer.

Minerals: the government's recommendation of 375 mg for **magnesium** is fine, but assumes we can get all that from food and absorb it all. In practice we lose vast amounts of magnesium through stress. The most important thing in choosing a magnesium supplement is what the magnesium is combined with (all minerals have to be combined with something). Magnesium carbonate and magnesium oxide are pretty useless. Far more effective (because better absorbed) are magnesium citrate or magnesium fumarate, magnesium malate or magnesium gluconate, or magnesium chelated (combined) with an amino acid, e.g. magnesium taurate, magnesium bisglycinate.

Regarding **zinc**, the government's recommendation of 10 mg per day is not quite enough for most of us these days. I would suggest 15 mg per day, and that is what most supplements provide. Zinc is drained out of our systems by the toxic metals like nickel, cadmium and mercury that surround us in an industrialised environment.

There are dizzying numbers of supplement companies out there, with a new one popping up every minute, so that even professional nutritional practitioners can't really keep up. I recommend products by about 20 different companies (and have absolutely no commercial or financial links with any of them). One useful criterion, as well as the issues discussed above about minimal junk and maximum nutrient content, is: do they have a technical department, staffed by nutritional therapists, that you can phone up and ask for advice? They should have.

At the time of writing (summer 2019), my favourites in the UK are:

- Viridian (very pure, very ethical, and their Vitamin D and Vitamin K come in really tiny capsules)

- Metabolics (very pure, very knowledgeable, very informative catalogue)

- Pure Bio (no junk) and BioCare (particularly good for liquid minerals, vitamins B and C, assorted gut treatments and children's products)

- Nordic Naturals (a Scandinavian company that specialises in fish oils).

There are a great number of good firms in the USA, including ARG (Allergy Research Group), Biotics, BodyBio, Jarrow and Life Extension, and they have a vast range of supplements. My favourite American firms in terms of purity (i.e. no junk) are Pure Encapsulations and Seeking Health.

I must stress, all this is only AT TIME OF WRITING. It is a field that changes fast. At any moment, a new and even better company might pop up. And more worryingly, at any moment a currently-very-good company could get bought up/taken over by a pharmaceutical firm or other corporation – it does happen – and the next thing you know, they're increasing their profits by stuffing the capsules with chalk (calcium carbonate). So this advice can only be a snapshot; don't take it as gospel, but DO take your magnifying glass to the health-food shop!

Choosing probiotics

The same principles apply. Here it really is a case of "more is more". You want at least 10 billion viable organisms, i.e. lots of living friendly bacteria. The greater the numbers, the greater the chance that some of them will hang around and take root. It's a bit like scattering seeds. Most of them won't "take", so you need to maximise the chances. Look for a wide range of species of Lactobacillus, (e.g. L. Acidophilus, L. Rhamnosus, L. Plantarum, L. Bulgaricus and more), and some Bifidobacterium species such as Bifidobacterium Longum, Bifido bifidum, and Bifido breve. Bifido infantis is particularly helpful in new babies who for one reason or another aren't being breastfed, and in those babies who were unfortunately given antibiotics at or soon after birth.

Multi-vitamins and multi-minerals

If they are top quality, these may be useful as a stop-gap measure for a while. But they have several drawbacks. Firstly, they may contain incompatible elements. For example, if they have both zinc and iron, the iron will stop the zinc being fully absorbed. And if they have both calcium and magnesium, the calcium will stop the magnesium being fully absorbed. Secondly, if they contain Vitamin A, there is a risk of overdosing on Vitamin A if you take them for a long period. Thirdly, they usually don't contain enough of anything to make a significant difference.

Supplements for children

Beware supplements disguised as sweeties – they may in fact be sweeties disguised as supplements. Watch out for sugar, artificial sweeteners and artificial colourings. Healthy kids don't need supplements anyway, they need good food, more sunshine and less screen time. Poorly kids **may** need supplements, and nutritional practitioners find that what most unwell children are lacking is zinc, magnesium, the B vitamins and Vitamin D. Sometimes iodine and Vitamin C as well, particularly in those who keep going down with infections. A few drops of the relevant nutrient in water (or **very** dilute fruit juice if really necessary) may do the trick. With kids who are fussy/faddy eaters, some zinc drops daily for a few weeks can sometimes work wonders – they may even start eating broccoli without bribery! And a good kiddies' probiotics can often sort out a tendency to tummy ache and diarrhoea/constipation. But of course you must consult a health professional if your child is persistently unwell.

How to introduce supplements?

The principle of "Suck it and See" applies to supplements as well as foods. Always introduce new supplements one at a time, i.e. one new one per day, to be sure it agrees with you.

What times of day to take supplements?

A good basic schedule is:

With Breakfast: B complex, Vitamin C, probiotic.

With Dinner: Zinc, Magnesium, Vitamin D.

I've almost given up suggesting supplements at lunchtime because no one can remember them!

(There is lots more info about Vitamins C and D in Chapter 1, Winter.)

For how long to keep taking them?

Vitamins B and C, probiotics and probably magnesium, can be taken indefinitely if you find they help. But with all other minerals, and with the fat-soluble vitamins and essential fatty acids (omegas 3 and 6), it is possible to overdose. So either get yourself tested (at Biolab or TDL) or take them only seasonally, as described in Chapters 1–4.

What will my GP think about all this?

Older doctors like myself had just one hour of nutrition teaching in a six-year course (and that was all about extreme deficiency states). Newly qualified doctors today tell me they still only have between three and eight hours of such training. This was confirmed recently on Radio 4's Food Programme, where two student doctors described their heroic efforts to try and get nutrition onto the medical school timetable in a meaningful way.[170]

Nutrition is simply applied biochemistry. We learn lots of biochemistry in medical school, but we don't learn what it is for; most doctors forget it within a couple of years, because they haven't used it – they weren't taught how to apply it. They think nutrition is just fluffy "lifestyle" medicine, and don't realise that there is a vast amount of hard science behind it.

If your GP is open and interested, you could invite them to check out the British Society for Ecological Medicine (www.bsem.

org.uk), which trains GPs and other doctors in Nutritional and Environmental Medicine. The "Environmental" bit is the subject of the next and final chapter. You might even buy them a copy of this book – if they can find the time to read it.

CHAPTER 7

TOX/
DETOX

You Can't Poison the Planet Without Poisoning the People

What's in this chapter:

Introduction To Toxicity

The impact of artificial chemicals on our bodies is immense, and really requires a whole book to itself. In this chapter I will be able to give only an outline of the problem and its solutions, but I hope it will encourage you to find out more, ask questions, and begin to think about how you can protect yourself, your family and our planet.

The first thing to say is that good nutrition is the single most important way to protect yourself against toxic chemicals. Vitamins and minerals help keep toxins out, and they also help your liver to get rid of those which do get through.[171]

The second thing is to remember that there are seven **de**toxification methods you can use to get rid of these toxins, and they are coming up on pages 297–307. So if you find the information that follows, about the chemicals to which we are exposed daily, a bit daunting or depressing, do remember: there is light at the end of this tunnel. Some people might want to skip over my bullet-point lists of toxins, and the other information, and go straight to the "Detox" section that begins on page 294; that's fair enough. On the other hand, knowing the dangers we face can also be empowering, because once armed with the facts, we can do something about them, both for ourselves and for others. And in each section about toxic chemicals, I have tried to suggest alternatives we can use, where they exist, and/or nutrients which get rid of those toxins.

So much for the health warning: now strap in, hold your nerve and hold your nose!

To get a sense of perspective, let's start with an approximate timescale:

- 3.5 billion years ago – life began on earth

- 600 million years ago – first multi-cellular life forms

- 200 million years ago – first mammals

- 15 million years ago – first great apes

- 2 million years ago – first human species

- 200,000 years ago – first modern Homo sapiens

- 10,000 years ago – the Agricultural Revolution began

- 200–250 years ago – the Industrial Revolution began

- 50–150 years ago – modern diseases like cancer, heart disease and Alzheimer's started to become epidemics (as opposed to rarities). They began earlier in those countries that industrialised early, like the UK, and later in those where industrialisation came later.

Since the Industrial Revolution we have synthesised 80,000–100,000 artificial chemicals. They are in our soil, food, water and air. We therefore eat them, inhale them and touch them, so they are in our bodies and brains. Most of them are lipophilic, so they dissolve in our cell membranes, which are largely made of lipids (fats), and thereby enter every body system. So they can cause symptoms in any and every part of the body and brain.[172,173] Our detox systems are not evolved to deal with them, but some people cope better than others, because of genetic differences in liver detox enzyme capacity.

Before considering some of these chemicals and what they do to us, there are a few general concepts we will need to understand:

- **Acute** vs **chronic** toxicity. "Acute" means a one-off obvious poisoning episode. "Chronic" refers to cumulative exposure to low levels over many years.

- **Safe levels**. The media and even learned journals talk about "safe levels" of toxins. But the only really safe level of a poison is zero.

- **Proof**. You will sometimes read reports saying there is no conclusive "proof" that substance X does any harm. But the concept of "proof" as generally used in medicine does not quite apply when considering toxicity. In a drug trial, you need "absolute proof" that a drug is safe and effective. But to obtain absolute proof that a synthetic chemical is harmful would be neither practical nor ethical. Hence what we need to apply is the Precautionary Principle (see below), a basic tenet of safe medical practice.

- **The cocktail effect**. We are never exposed to just one or two chemicals, but to a whole cocktail of them. The effects of this cocktail can never be safely or accurately or ethically evaluated in conventional studies.

- **Total load**. In assessing a person's level of toxicity, we have to consider the "total load" on their system, including: how many toxins? Which ones? How much of each? In which body compartments? How are they affecting the immune system? The other systems? How are these toxicities interacting with possible nutrient deficiencies, gut function, exercise level, social/psychological stress etc?

- **The Precautionary Principle**. If it looks as if it's poisonous, it probably is. If it has made some people ill, it may make others ill. If it's a molecule that doesn't occur in nature, or a metal that belongs in the earth's crust but not in our bodies, then it probably doesn't fit well with our biochemistry. If it's toxic to some living things, it may well be toxic to other living things. If in doubt, leave it out.

And a couple more points before we go on to discuss specific substances:

- **Age** is very important. The younger you are, the more dangerous synthetic chemicals are to you. The foetus is most at risk, the grandparent least. This is because exposure to synthetic chemicals, like exposure to radiation, can damage DNA. Today's children are more at risk of mental and physical damage from toxins than any previous generation.

And it's not just synthetics. **Natural substances** produced by moulds and some bacteria can be just as toxic as artificial chemicals, and can cause similar problems. And we need to be careful what we mean by "natural"; heavy metals are natural in that they occur naturally in the earth's crust, but they become toxic when mined and smelted and changed by industrial processing. They are only totally safe if we leave them under the ground. Same with crude oil.

Which Toxic Chemicals Are We Talking About?

There is no totally satisfactory way to categorise 80,000+ substances. It is perhaps simplest to divide them into elements and compounds, and to divide the elements into the two major categories that cause us problems, namely heavy metals and halogens.

The **heavy metals** that can affect us include aluminium, antimony, arsenic, beryllium, cadmium, lead, mercury, nickel, thallium, titanium, tin and more; we will only describe the sources and effects of five of them.

The toxic **halogens** are fluorine, chlorine and bromine.

The synthetic compounds fall into numerous sub-categories, but we'll just look at some of them, based mostly on where we encounter them in our day-to-day lives.

But before we go into a little more detail about some of these toxic chemicals and what they can do to us, let's meet someone who was directly affected by toxicity as a result of his job: an example of a still-not-fully-recognised occupational illness.

Case History: Graham's Aerotoxic Syndrome

Graham was a pilot, aged 49, and had been flying with a major international airline for 24 years. Among those like Graham who fly very frequently, for work, over many years, serious health problems are not uncommon.[174] Graham's story is typical of what I see in pilots and cabin crew, and also in some business people who fly once or twice a week.

Graham was totally fit and healthy for most of his life. His health problems had begun in an apparently minor way, 10 years before he came to see me. At that point he had been flying for 14 years, and began to notice that he was getting headaches at the end of a long flight. They would wear off within a few hours of landing. Then a couple of years later he began to experience some pain, numbness and tingling in his arms and hands, and the headaches became more severe and long-lasting, occurring both during and after flights. Brain scans found nothing abnormal, and the GP suggested painkillers.

Regarding the increasing numbness in his arms and hands, Graham saw a neurologist, a rheumatologist, an orthopaedic surgeon, a physiotherapist and a chiropractor. None of them found anything wrong. It became increasingly difficult for Graham to work. He was changed from long-haul flights to short-haul flights, but he then got even worse (we'll see why shortly).

The final straw came when Graham started to become cognitively impaired. His wife said he was "forgetting things, talking nonsense sometimes, and struggling to spell simple words". He was no longer reading, found conversation "terribly tiring", and would occasionally burst into tears without knowing why. He also had some numbness in one foot now; again, the neurologist et al. did not know why.

By the time Graham came to see me he had been retired on ill-health grounds for nearly three years. "I should have stopped sooner," he told me. "Really, that last year, I already couldn't think straight. I shouldn't have been in the cockpit. It wasn't just the headaches, it was like a thick blanket of fog around my brain, slowing down all my reflexes. It still is."

This phenomenon occurring in airline pilots has been researched and documented by Dr Sarah McKenzie Ross.[175] Remember, to be accepted onto a pilots' training course, you have to be not just fit and healthy but very bright. Dr McKenzie Ross's studies have confirmed serious loss of mental ability in a large sample of pilots, all of whom started off as people with an impressively high IQ.[176]

Graham's symptoms were, typically, in his central nervous system. Many pilots and cabin crew also have symptoms in their respiratory systems, digestive systems and other body systems as well. Some pilots and cabin crew call it "plane flu".

Since his forced early retirement, Graham's wife had had him on a very pure diet, high in antioxidant-rich fruit and vegetables. She felt this had prevented further deterioration, and possibly improved him a little. He wasn't sure; all he knew was that he was miserable, disabled and unemployed, with no explanation.

On testing, all Graham's nutrients except zinc were at good

levels. But we did find some toxic substances in his body, including an organophosphate (OP) insecticide and an extraordinarily high level of the toxic metal, nickel. These chemicals and many others are found in the air on aeroplanes, both in the cockpit where the pilot sits and in the cabin where the passengers and cabin crew are. Many of them are found in polluted urban air too – but on a plane they're more concentrated, you can't get away and you can't open a window.

The on-board toxic chemical that has caused most concern is Tri-Cresyl Phosphate (TCP), a type of Organo-Phosphate (OP) used as an "anti-wear additive" in the engine oil.[177] Unfortunately, the air supply on all passenger jet aircraft (except the Boeing 787) comes into the passenger cabin and the cockpit from the engines, unfiltered. This air (known as "bleed air" as it is bled off the engine compression section) gets contaminated with heated engine oils. These contain hundreds of different chemicals, including TCP, which are therefore present in the air that passengers and cabin crew and pilots are breathing.[178] This leakage is usually slight, but it can sometimes be extreme, so the toxic gases can actually be smelt ("smelly socks" smell) and even occasionally seen (a white mist) – this is a "fume event".

TCP is dangerous to us because, like other OPs, it inhibits the enzyme acetyl cholinesterase, which has the job of deconstructing the neurotransmitter acetyl choline when it has done its job. So we get an unnatural build-up of acetyl choline in the synaptic space between two nerve cells, leading to nerve cell damage, numbness and eventually paralysis. TCP has been found in the blood and the clothing of people just stepping off a plane, but it was three years since Graham had been near a plane. The TCP would have disappeared; not necessarily from his body, but certainly from his blood and other accessible body fluids. As a highly fat-soluble toxin it may well have been hiding in fatty tissue (including the brain), or it may have done its damage and gone; there is as yet no reliable way to test this.

However, I did find another OP, the insecticide para-DiChloroBenzene, in Graham's fat cells (at that time I was able to order a fat biopsy, a test which now hardly exists in the UK). Insecticides are sprayed inside the plane when travelling to or from a tropical country. Para-DiChloroBenzene is nasty stuff,[179] but is used very commonly as a moth-killer in people's homes. (See page 289 for safe, natural alternatives.) It is not possible to be certain that this is what was sprayed on any or all of the many trips that Graham flew; cabin crew with similar illnesses often cannot tell me which insecticide they sprayed in the cabin last week, still less years ago. But these substances last a very long time.

The other toxin I found in Graham's system was nickel. The engine's rapidly moving parts contain nickel or nickel alloys, and tiny (nano-) particles of nickel may fly off and find their way into the cabin air and cockpit air, again because of defective seals between the engine and the rest of the plane. I find this metal at very high levels in pilots and cabin crew.

Remember that Graham got markedly worse when he was changed from long-haul flights to short-haul flights? On short-haul flights, a higher proportion of his time was spent in take-off and landing. This means more fumes from the other planes on the tarmac; the engine is sucking in diesel exhaust fumes from the plane in front, just like in a traffic jam. And take-off and landing are also when the majority of fume events occur. Airlines acknowledge that these fume events occur "occasionally", but my patients who are pilots or cabin crew think they happen more often than that.

As well as insecticides, TCP and nickel, other substances that may be in the air in aeroplanes include the neurotoxin toluene (out-gassing from the in-flight magazines), thallium from onboard computers, beryllium in some engine bearings, mould from air-conditioning systems, benzene and nitrosamines from burnt fuel, anti-freeze for de-icing the outside of the plane in very cold conditions (it gets into the engine and thus into the air inside the plane), styrene gas from polystyrene meal trays and seats and insulation, poly-brominated biphenyls (PBBs) used as fire retardants, and plasticisers like phthalates which are oestrogenic endocrine disruptors – as are the OP insecticides and TCP, which may account for the increased rate of breast cancer reported by female pilots and cabin staff.[180]

Graham was willing to do everything possible to get the neurotoxins out of his body, and his wife was willing to support him. I put him on the detoxification regime described on pages 297–307, sweating out the toxins in the sauna, making and drinking fresh organic green vegetable juice every morning, and taking the herbal remedy milkthistle to support his liver.[181] I also gave him Vitamin C, zinc and an amino acid called methionine, all of which help to remove nickel. Graham's zinc level was low, despite a good diet, and all other nutrients were normal. Nickel pushes out zinc, and giving the patient zinc "pushes back", pushing out the nickel as well as eventually normalising the zinc level.

Graham turned out to have a slight genetic weakness in his PON1 gene, reducing his ability to detoxify OP-type chemicals.[182]

What made him ill, though, was the chemical exposure, not the gene. In pre-industrial times, someone with his genetic constitution (and it is not uncommon) would have been no more at risk of illness than anyone else. Occasionally, very chemically sensitive people will become ill after a one-off fume event on a plane. But the type of chronic illness that Graham suffered is what's meant by the phrase "Aerotoxic Syndrome". Most air-crew have both chronic exposure AND periodic acute exposure from fume events. The "acute on chronic" effect can make them very, very ill.

Graham stuck to his regime and recovery was slow. After six months his cognitive abilities were improving; he could read a newspaper but not yet a book. His numb and tingling limbs were no better, so I added a high dose vitamin B12 which helps the nerve cells to heal. Within a few weeks he was noticing an improvement, and I sent him to a cranial osteopath who also helped. Although Graham's diet was good, he needed to add in a lot more healthy fats; the brain and nervous system are largely made of fats. So I made sure he was having plenty of oily fish, avocado, nuts and seeds, plus hemp oil (raw), coconut oil (to cook with) and olive oil. I also gave him both omega 3 and omega 6 supplements for a while, and some phosphatidyl choline. Also known as PC, this is made from sunflower lecithin or soya lecithin. It is a natural component of our cell membranes, a gentle aid to liver detox and a great restorer of brain function. It is particularly helpful when someone has been poisoned with a lipophilic (fat-soluble) chemical.[183]

After another year, Graham was improved further, and his memory and concentration were approaching normal. Two years on, he was able to start thinking of looking for a job, although not in the airline industry. The numbness and tingling is gone from the foot and one arm and hand but not quite from the other, and returns if he gets overtired. He will never be completely better.

Graham was lucky in that his symptoms were only in one system of the body. More usually, frequent flyers who get sick have symptoms in **every** system of the body. This is because most of the chemicals involved are "lipophilic": they dissolve in fat. Our cell membranes are largely made of fat, so these chemicals pass through them and get distributed to every part of the body. One unfortunate consequence of having symptoms in every system of the body is that your overworked and overwhelmed GP may well dismiss the whole lot as "psychological". Certainly, Aerotoxic Syndrome has psychological **consequences**; there are poisons in the brain, and they can make some people slightly crazy. And being both ill and misunderstood will make anybody depressed eventually. But it's not imagination. Pilots like Graham are bright, ambitious people who adore their work, and are devastated when they realise what it's doing to them.

Aerotoxic Syndrome is a hotly contested diagnosis. The airline industry still says it does not exist, although they have surprisingly high numbers of staff off sick at any one time, there is an increased prevalence of cancer among airline staff,[184] and there have been many unexplained deaths of young pilots and cabin crew. Some of these deaths have been recorded by ex-cabin crew member Dee Passon, at the website www.angelfleet.net. The existence of Aerotoxic Syndrome is disputed in much the same way that asbestos was considered to be safe and tobacco was claimed to be harmless in the relatively recent past. And it hasn't reached the medical textbooks yet, much as ME/Chronic Fatigue Syndrome had not done 20 years ago, being regularly dismissed as a psychological concoction or "Yuppie Flu".

But the evidence is accumulating and it won't go away.[185,186,187] There is the clinical evidence of patients like Graham, seen by myself and colleagues over recent years. And there is also a growing body of scientific research. As an example, Professor Mohammed Abou-Donia of Duke University in North Carolina found that after 45 hours of flying over a period of 10 days, a pilot's level of antibodies against his own brain proteins increased, and the increase correlated with the impairment of his cognitive function. We shouldn't be making antibodies against our own tissues **at all**! Such autoimmune responses are often a reaction to chemical toxicity.[188]

How often have you heard yourself or someone else say, straight after a plane trip: "I feel rotten; I must have caught a bug from the person I sat next to on the flight"? Well, bugs don't cause symptoms that quickly; infections take time to incubate. It might not be flu at all; it might just be a response to all the unpleasant chemicals you've been breathing in on the plane. It helps to take loads of Vitamin C on the flight. And you can also make flying a bit safer for yourself as a passenger, by getting a "sky mask" from www.angelfleet.net – the times you are most likely to need it are at take-off and landing, as above.

And now let's do a brief and inevitably somewhat simplified survey of the toxins we may all encounter in the course of our ordinary lives, whatever our occupation.

Heavy Metals – Environmental Sources And Biological Effects

Mercury

Sources: Mercury is found in "silver" amalgam dental fillings, tuna fish, broken thermometers, industrial effluent, and in old vaccination stocks in the form of "Thimerosal".

Effects: Neurological and psychiatric symptoms,[189,190] bleeding gums, metallic taste in mouth, gut disorders, tinnitus, autoimmune disease and more.

Lead

Sources: Old house paint, old pipes, cosmetics – especially skin whiteners, imported toys, factory emissions, coal burning and more.

Effects: Gut ache, bowel problems, nausea and vomiting, developmental delay, impulsivity/aggression,[191,192] memory and learning problems, muscular weakness/fatigue, insomnia, anaemia, Alzheimer's-like pathology, and more.

Nickel

Sources: Stainless-steel pots and pans (stainless steel is 14 per cent nickel), coins, orthodontic appliances, cheap jewellery, margarine, cigarette smoke, batteries, electroplating, fossil fuel combustion, car exhaust fumes (actually virtually all the toxic metals have been found in diesel/petrol exhaust).

Effects: Cancer,[193,194] especially of breast and lung, hypoglycaemia, zinc deficiency, manganese deficiency, skin sensitivity/nickel allergy, endocrine (hormone) disruption, diseases of heart, kidney and immune system.

Aluminium

Sources: Deodorants/anti-perspirants, aluminium pots and pans, as an adjuvant in some vaccinations, cooking/wrapping food in "tin" foil, some antacid medications, aluminium drink cans, take-away containers, cosmetics.

Effects: Dementia/Alzheimer's in adults, neurological damage/delay in children,[195] breast cancer,[196] autoimmunity, kidney/liver/bone damage, heart/lung damage, endocrine disruption, DNA damage.

Cadmium

Sources: Tobacco smoke, burning of fossil fuels and tyres, yellow paint (including artists' paint), some fertilisers, toys, cosmetics, some soya-based baby milks, carpet underlay.

Effects: Bone pain and bone damage,[197] multi-organ damage, headaches, hair loss, endocrine disruption, gynaecological cancers and pancreatic cancer,[198] zinc deficiency.

It is very useful to think of these toxic metals (and toxins in general) as "**anti-nutrients**", a concept for which I am indebted to Dr John McLaren-Howard, a brilliant scientist and long-term mentor to many in the BSEM. For example, nickel and cadmium displace zinc, mercury displaces sulphur and selenium, aluminium displaces silicon, and excess copper will displace zinc. Conversely, on the plus side, zinc is useful to get rid of nickel and cadmium, selenium and zinc help get rid of mercury, and silicon (as silica) helps get rid of aluminium. But not on their own – see "detox methods" on pages 297–307).

Mercury toxicity – the hazards of common metal dental fillings

Many of us have grey metal fillings in our mouths. Sometimes known as "silver" fillings, dentists call them "amalgam" fillings, and they contain mostly the neurotoxic metal mercury, along with smaller amounts of tin, silver and copper. The mercury in fillings has been shown to leak out[199,200] and to reach all parts of the body,[201] and is implicated in neurological diseases.[202,203,204]

Before you can remove the mercury from your system by the detoxification methods described later in this chapter, you would need to have any amalgam fillings **safely** changed over to white fillings by a specialist dentist, a member of the International Academy of Oral Medicine and Toxicology (IAOMT). These dentists use methods that minimise the release of mercury into your body while drilling, and that is vital.

Some people choose to do this for purely preventive reasons, perhaps because of a family history of dementia or Parkinson's Disease. Others do it because they themselves are suffering from a neurological disease like Multiple Sclerosis, and have high mercury levels.

Toxic Halogens/Halides – Environmental Sources And Biological Effects

The halogens are fluorine, chlorine, bromine and iodine. They are called by these names when they are in their elemental form, i.e. as atoms. When they react with another substance and gain an electron, they become ions, and are then called the halides: fluoride, chloride, bromide and iodide. Fluorine is highly toxic in both forms, i.e. as fluorine and fluoride. Bromine and bromide are also both toxic. Chlor**ine** is toxic, whereas chlor**ide** is a vital part of our biochemistry. And iodine and iodide, in contrast, are both essential to our bodies, so although they come into the category of halogen/halide, they are not toxic except, like any other substance, in massive overdose.

The breast and prostate tissues need iod**ine**, whereas the thyroid and the skin require iod**ide**.[205] All the other body tissues need and use both iodine and iodide. One of the main problems with the toxic halogens/halides is that they push iodine/iodide out of the body, acting as anti-nutrients, and are therefore implicated in our population's widespread iodine deficiency and in diseases of the thyroid, prostate and breast, among others. The positive flip side of this is that the best way to get the toxic halogens/halides out of your body is to take a combination of iodine and iodide, such as Iodoral, Iodizyme or Lugol's iodine.

Sources of the toxic halogens/halides:

They may come from other chemicals, e.g. compounds such as pesticides, dioxins, CFCs and many prescription drugs and over-the-counter drugs. The main environmental sources of specific toxic halogens/halides are as follows:

Fluoride
This is added to tap water in the West Midlands, parts of north-east England and Cumbria, Cheshire and a few other areas, and in the Republic of Ireland. It is also found in most toothpastes, dental

drops, fissure sealants and some mouthwashes. It is in many asthma inhalers, and other drugs, and is in the non-stick coating of non-stick pans. Check the label – where you see the prefix "flu" it indicates the presence of fluoride in the molecule. Why is there so much of it about? Short answer: it's a by-product of the phosphate fertiliser industry, which had a major waste disposal problem with fluoride, until they convinced various health and dental authorities in the USA (but not in continental Europe) to put it in the drinking water.

Chlorine

This is put in our tap water and swimming pools as a disinfectant/ antibacterial. It's also in bleach, PVC plastic and bleached wood-pulp and is released from many of the compounds mentioned above. Chlorine from tap water gets into us not just by drinking it and cooking with it, but also via the skin and lungs when showering or bathing.

You can get a plumbed-in **water filter** from the Fresh Water Filter Company or Silverline or any other reputable water-filter company. They should be able to talk you through exactly what the filter does and does not remove. They are better than one that sits on the worktop, because they enable you to use safe, filtered water for cooking and making hot drinks as well as for drinking directly. And you don't want your filtered water sitting in a plastic jug in a warm kitchen; you'd be drinking the plasticiser chemicals.

Bromine/bromide

This is in some drugs, flame retardants (PBBs), insecticides, fumigants, dyes, and soft drinks. At one point it was added to bread in the USA!

And now to the biological damage that they do:

Effects of the toxic halogens:

Fluoride
- Damages structure of bone by following calcium into bone cells (see page 229, and refs 153 and 154)

- Increases incidence of primary bone cancer, osteosarcoma[206]

- Damages kidneys[207]

- Interferes with nerve signal transmission, affects brain function[208]

- Damages thyroid gland

- Damages pineal gland, interferes with synthesis of melatonin

- Brings aluminium and other toxic metals with it

- Replaces hydrogen bonds in DNA, leading to foetal damage

- Increases oxidative stress and lipid peroxidation

- Damages enzymes by attaching to metal ions at active sites on the enzyme

- Interferes with the G proteins which facilitate messages across cell membranes

Chlorine

Chlorine in our tap water has been linked with:

- Colon cancer[209]

- Bladder cancer

- Asthma[210]

- Eczema and dry, irritated skin

- Heart disease/atherosclerosis

- Infertility, miscarriages, birth defects

Some of these effects may be because chlorine in tap water combines with natural substances to form Tri-Halo-Methanes (THMs) such as **Chloroform**. These are also called disinfection by-products (DBPs).

Bromine/bromide

- Cognitive and behavioural disorders (it used to be used as a sedative)

- Reproductive dysfunction – infertility[211]

- Lung damage

- Kidney damage

- Brain damage

- Corrosive – irritant to eyes, skin and mucous membranes

- Slow healing

- Acne

- Headaches

- Gut disorders and anorexia

- Thyroid disorders (possibly by displacing iodine)

- Cardiovascular disorders

- Joint pains

Remember, though, taking iodine/iodide, combined with the detox methods on pages 297–307, will help to get these toxic halogens/halides out of your system.

Synthetic Compounds – Environmental Sources And Biological Effects

These compounds include – take a deep breath:

- Air pollutants, both outdoors and indoors

- Biocides – pesticides, herbicides (weed-killers), fungicides, insecticides

- Plastics and plasticisers

- Personal care products

- Perfumes

- Hair products

- Laundry chemicals

- Building materials

- Decorating materials

- Paints, varnishes, glues

- Domestic cleaning chemicals

- Detergents and disinfectants

🌿 Drugs

🌿 Food additives

Many of them contain substances which are classified by the World Health Organization (WHO) and other concerned organisations as carcinogens, teratogens or Endocrine Disrupting Compounds (EDCs). Many are neurotoxins. And many are Persistent Organic Pollutants, or POPs; they are still found in our soil and our bodies decades after being banned (yes, some of them do get banned. And don't be confused by the use of the word "organic"; it has a different meaning here. In chemistry it simply means any substance containing carbon. Some of the most toxic substances known are "organic" in that technical sense. In this context it has nothing to do with your healthy, pesticide-free vegetables!)

Dry-cleaning fluids – another hazard!
The dry-cleaning process uses chemicals like trichloroethylene and tetrachloroethylene (or perchloroethylene – 'perc'). The International Agency for Research on Cancer (IARC) has found them to be carcinogenic in mammals.[212] We are mammals. Best to avoid dry-cleaning, but if you have to, at least do it in summer, when you can hang the dry-cleaned items on the line outside for a couple of days to "out-gas" before bringing them into your house.

Outdoor air pollutants

These do include pesticides, dioxins from fires and assorted factory gases, but are mostly from traffic fumes, which contain:

✍ Carbon monoxide and dioxide

✍ Nitric oxide and nitrogen dioxide

✍ Sulphur dioxide

✍ Pentanes and hexanes

✍ Benzene, toluene and Polycyclic Aromatic Hydrocarbons (PAHs)

✍ Ozone (from action of sunlight on hydrocarbons)

✍ Nitrosamines

✍ Particulate matter (PM) from diesel exhaust

The WHO says that particulate matter (PM) from diesel exhaust affects more people than any other pollutant, contributing to numerous serious illnesses. These include deaths from lung cancer,[213] heart attacks,[214] strokes, and kidney and bladder disease. PM is also implicated in neurodegenerative disease such as Alzheimer's occurring in young adults and even in children.[215] One study has even shown that sleep disruption in pre-school children is linked with exposure to PM pollution from when they were in the womb.[216]

Nitrogen dioxide is associated with deaths from colon cancer and PM pollution with deaths from kidney and bladder cancers.[217] Nitrogen dioxide causes Chronic Obstructive Pulmonary Disease (COPD).[218] And nitrogen dioxide and PM pollution together have been linked to autistic spectrum disorders in children (see refs 134 and 135). Sulphur dioxide exposure has been linked with migraine[219] and childhood asthma,[220] and benzene exposure with very many diseases.[221] Neurodegenerative diseases have been linked with ozone[222] and with toluene,[223] and the PAHs with oesophageal cancer[224] and – again – childhood asthma.[225]

The nitrosamines (from cigarette smoke as well as car fumes) have been linked to breast cancer,[226] stomach cancer and generally to damage to our DNA.[227] And air pollution in general has been linked to inflammation, atherosclerosis, multi-organ damage, childhood leukaemia, reduced cognitive function, diabetes, allergic rhinitis, autoimmune disease, osteoporosis and fractures, conjunctivitis, dry-eye disease, blepharitis, inflammatory bowel disease, increased blood-clotting, poorer kidney function, eczema, urticaria, acne and skin ageing.

There are hundreds of studies showing the damaging effects of air pollution on our mental and physical health; more are appearing every week. I am very grateful to the researcher and lecturer Dr Rachel Nicoll, who has an encyclopaedic knowledge of this topic, for pointing me in the direction of some of these studies. She also notes that among the now huge number of studies, there are some showing no effects of pollutants on our health. These tend to be the earlier studies, done before we had more accurate ways of measuring pollution, or adequate understanding of the many ways in which we can accumulate it in our bodies. And some of these early studies only considered exposure from one source, not taking into account the fact we may be exposed to a particular toxin from many sources (e.g. food, water and skin contact as well as air). And of course almost no study design can fully allow for the "cocktail" effect, the fact that we are exposed to dozens of different toxins every day.

Action to protect ourselves and our children from the effects of outdoor air pollution has to be collective as well as individual. Yes, we all need to drive less. But only by pressuring government to create clean, cheap and reliable public transport, and industry to reduce the production of toxic petrol, diesel and other fossil fuels, will we be able to breathe our way safely into the future.

When it comes to indoor pollution, however there is much more we can do on an individual level.

Indoor air pollutants

These include toxins like formaldehyde, solvents and other Volatile Organic Compounds (VOCs) which "out-gas" from all sorts of things inside our houses.[228] The sources include building materials, paint, varnish, chipboard, carpets, carpet glue, furniture polish, grout and sealants, as well as the fire-retardants[229] in new mattresses, sofas, curtains and carpets. And dry-cleaning chemicals. And moth balls (they are insecticide). And domestic detergents and cleaning chemicals, laundry chemicals, stain-removers. And in old houses, asbestos and lead. And "air-freshener". I once stopped a patient's migraines just by persuading her to throw out the air-freshener. (It's rarely that simple). And moulds – see pages 129–130. Open the windows!

There are alternatives to most of these polluting indoor substances. Ecos, Auro and Graphenstone make safe paints. You can have hard floors and rugs instead of chemical-impregnated carpets. You can use safe laundry and household cleaning products from Suma, Ecover and similar companies. You can use lavender oil instead of moth balls, or you can get safe, lavender-based sprays from Greenfibres, which do the job as well as moth balls without poisoning you. You can use natural essential oils for perfuming yourself and your home. Most importantly, when you need a new mattress, you can get an organic one; it won't contain any pesticides or other toxins; it won't have that "new mattress smell" when you unwrap it.

Mattresses – what's in them?

I have had a few patients who became ill shortly after buying a new mattress. Most mattresses contain flame retardants and other synthetic chemicals. These chemicals "out-gas" from the mattress, and during the night the person is inhaling them, as well as potentially absorbing them through the skin. Some people can cope with this; others can't. A more chemically sensitive person is likely to be able to smell the chemicals, whereas their sleeping partner may not; genetic difference again. If you need a new mattress, it's best to buy an organic one from somewhere like Abaca. Abaca are in Wales and they deliver all over the UK. You can call them on 01269 598491.

There is more on how to make your home safer on pages 164–167. And much excellent information on all this is to be found in chapter 19 of *Environmental Medicine in Clinical Practice* – see the Resources section at the end of the book.

Indoor water pollutants

What's coming out of your tap? The water companies have processes that remove bacteria, but they do not remove heavy metals, pesticide residues and other chemical pollutants, and they add chlorine and in some areas fluoride. Nor do they remove antibiotics peed out onto the fields by (non-organic) farm animals, which will seep into reservoirs. What goes around comes around. They also don't remove traces of synthetic hormones. What are traces of synthetic hormones doing in our water? They are peed out by all the women using HRT, or the contraceptive pill, or the hormonal IUCD (coil). Or by farm animals injected with hormones, a practice which is illegal in the EU, but may become legal in the UK when/if we leave the EU.

Get a plumbed-in water filter: see page 275.

Personal care products

🌿 Conventional soap, shower gel, shampoo and conditioner

🌿 Deodorant, anti-perspirant, aftershave, perfume

🌿 Moisturiser, sunscreen, after-sun cream

You can get much safer versions of most of the above in good health-food shops; Suma make especially lovely safe soaps. Green People and Urtekram are good, safe brands too, at time of writing.

🌿 Bubble bath – use essential oils in the bath instead, like geranium, jasmine, rose, lavender or frankincense. They don't make bubbles but they do make nice smells

- Make-up, make-up remover – there are some slightly safer "mineral" versions, but I've not been that impressed when I've looked at the ingredients lists of most of them

- Nail varnish, nail varnish remover (if you must, please put it on outdoors. It's not a problem once it's on your nails and dry; the problem is inhaling it while you apply it)

- Hair dye, hair straightener, hair perming lotions, hair spray[230]

- Head lice treatments (see Chapter 3 for safe alternatives)

- Cosmetic implants: botox, silicone

- Tattoos, piercings – depending on the materials used

More about perfume
Most of the ingredients (listed and unlisted) are petrochemicals, not flower extracts. E.g:

- Parabens

- Phthalates

- Benzene

- Toluene

- Synthetic "musk"

These are endocrine disruptors, neurotoxins, carcinogens and teratogens. They are absorbed into our bodies through the skin and
through inhalation. Then there's:

- "Fragrance" or "Parfum" – like "flavouring" in a food, this can
  mean anything.

But perfumes and cosmetics generally, like processed foods, have
an ingredients list. So you can tell what's in them, right?

Wrong. Because there are loopholes in the law, meaning they
don't have to put everything on the list. The Environmental
Working Group (EWG) in the USA found that the average perfume
has 14 **unlisted** ingredients![231]

And remember, what applies to perfumes applies also to scented
candles and to plug-in room-scenting devices too. Essential oils
are a much safer option, for perfuming both yourself and your
house/flat.

Biocides
Pesticides, herbicides, fungicides, insecticides. It's the same principle; they kill things. Biocides damage the nervous system,
reproductive system, respiratory system and more. I've seen many
patients who have developed serious illnesses after accidental
exposure, such as walking through a field or orchard that was
being sprayed, or spending time in a house which had just been
treated for a wasps' nest, an ant infestation or mice. They often
end up with severe, prolonged fatigue and extreme sensitivity to
all other chemicals. Not everyone will be affected this way, as we
all differ in our genetic ability to get these substances out of our

bodies. But avoidance is the best policy. See below for safe alternatives.

Some biocides which have long been banned in Western countries, such as the Organo-Chlorines DDT, DDE and Lindane, are in fact still around, and have been found in the fat of polar bears quite recently, giving the bears assorted health problems, including osteoporosis.[232] This is because they are POPs – Persistent Organic Pollutants – i.e. virtually indestructible. (PCBs, the PolyChlorinated Biphenyls which preceded PBBs as flame retardants, are also POPs, and still around, and have been found in the arctic bears as well.) Inexcusably, many of these biocides were exported to – dumped in – developing countries, when they were banned in the UK. I have found some of them at high levels in people from India and Africa.

I've also found these chemicals in fat samples from older people living in the UK. I found Lindane in one elderly lady who finally traced it back to the time she was treated for headlice as a child, 70 years previously. These substances are not called Persistent for nothing. And they are strongly linked to breast cancer and to Non-Hodgkins Lymphoma, according to the WHO.

Organo-Phosphate (OP) biocides have replaced the Organo-Chlorines, but are neurotoxic, carcinogenic and endocrine-disrupting. That's progress for you. More recent biocides include the following:

- Carbamates – similar effects to the OPs

- Pyrethroids – e.g. Permethrin – used as a household insecticide for wasps and ants, but they kill bees too, and in mammals (like us) they damage the respiratory system and are neurotoxic, carcinogenic and endocrine-disrupting

- Glyphosate – this is the main constituent of "Round-up", an over-the-counter weed-killer used on domestic lawns and your local park. Damages the placenta, causes endocrine disruption. The WHO agency IARC (International Agency for Cancer Research) considers it probably carcinogenic in humans[233]

- Para-DiChloro Benzene – this is an important one, because it's used so commonly as a moth-killer; it's in those purple moth balls. It is "reasonably anticipated to be a human carcinogen".[234] There are safe, natural alternatives such as lavender oil. You can get natural essential oil of lavender from a good health-food shop, or better still, Greenfibres of Totnes have a great range of safe anti-moth products for clothes and furniture, based on lavender and neem oils. You can order online, or call them on 01803 868001

There is a recipe for a safe, natural insect repellent on page 108. Neem powder kills many insects too, with no negative effect on humans or other mammals.

Plastics and plasticisers
As well as clogging up our precious oceans, these are poisoning us directly. You find them in:

- Plastic water bottles (worse in hot sun. The plasticisers go into the water)

- Clingfilm/plastic wrap

- Plastic bags, food packaging

- Plastic pipes, plastic jugs

- Plastic toys, plastic watch straps

- Everywhere!

They mostly contain **phthalates**,[235] also used to soften **PVC**, **P**oly**V**inyl **C**hloride. (Don't be misled by the "Chloride" bit in PVC; what's released, especially when it burns, is chlorine, not chloride.) They are all endocrine disruptors, implicated in the epidemic of breast cancer, and PVC is implicated in liver cancer too. Use glass bottles, protected by a padded container you can get from a camping shop. Or if that's not possible (schools tend not to allow them), then stainless steel will have to do. But only for water; fruit juice will leach the nickel out of the stainless steel. One of the worst plastic chemicals is BPA, which needs a section to itself:

BPA – BisPhenol A

This is an oestrogen mimic. It is found in PolyCarbonate plastics, paints, car exhaust, cigarette smoke, pesticides, PCBs, till receipts, dioxins released from incinerators, the lining of cans of food, drink and baby food, and until very recently in the teats of some baby bottles. It's an endocrine disruptor. It sits on oestrogen receptors and has oestrogenic effects: it feminises male animals, causes erectile dysfunction in male workers occupationally exposed to it, accelerates female puberty, contributes to the obesity epidemic and is implicated in breast and prostate disease. It's also neurotoxic, and experimentally it increased the rate of proliferation in the cells of neuroblastoma, a type of brain tumour. And it's been linked to asthma and heart disease. And it's not banned in the UK.

Dioxins

Also known as PolyChlorinated Dibenzo-Dioxins (PCDDs) and PolyChlorinated Dibenzo Furans (PCDFs), these are industrial by-products from making herbicides, from bleaching textiles and paper, from metal smelting and refining and from municipal incinerators. They were a contaminant of Agent Orange in Vietnam, and were released on a large scale at the Seveso disaster in Italy in 1976 (see pages 244–245). They have got into our soil, and they increase up the food chain, so are found more in meat, fish, shellfish and dairy products than in plants; yes, it's an argument in favour of veganism. The dioxins are fat-soluble and get through our cell membranes, so into all body systems.

Their biological effects include:

🌿 Immune system damage

🌿 Cancer

🌿 Chloracne

🌿 Endocrine disruption, leading to:
- Reproductive and developmental problems – foetal toxicity
- Endometriosis
- Diabetes
- Thyroid disease

Hair dyes

These chemicals include azo-dyes, naphthols, diamines and more; some 5,000+ compounds. Some contain nickel too. The scalp has a very good blood supply, with lots of blood vessels very near the surface, so most of what you put on the scalp gets absorbed into the body. These chemicals have been linked with breast cancer and bladder cancer,[236] and it remains an open question whether they may be linked with leukaemia and lymphoma. Pure henna is probably safe, but a lot of so-called organic hair dyes are not. Read the label, and look up any ingredients that are unfamiliar. And remember, the longer it lasts, the less natural it is.

Medical sources of toxins

These include:

- Drugs – prescribed, OTC and illegal

- Metabolites of drugs (i.e. what the body turns them into)

- Dental fillings, bridges, crowns etc. (mercury, tin, titanium)

- Orthodontic devices (nickel)

- Fluoride in dental fissure sealants etc. (see pages 145, 166, 274–275 and 276–277)

- Vaccinations (may include aluminium or mercury, polysorbate 80, sorbitol, formaldehyde, monosodium glutamate and others)

🖉 Orthopaedic implants

🖉 Silicone breast implants and Botox (usually cosmetic rather than strictly medical)

How Do Toxins Do Their Damage?

There are several mechanisms by which they can harm us by:

🖉 Acting as anti-nutrients (see page 272)

🖉 Occupying active sites on enzyme molecules

🖉 Occupying hormone receptor sites

🖉 Interfering with cell signalling

🖉 Causing abnormal protein formation and auto-immune reactions

🖉 Leading to production of even more toxic metabolites

🖉 Damaging DNA, altering gene expression

🖉 Damaging cell membrane structure

🖉 Promoting inflammation and oxidative damage to cells

Detoxification – How To Begin

"Detox" is an overused word these days. What I mean by it is seven specific methods for actively removing toxins from your body, and I will describe those methods. But in addition to active detoxification, you first need to do three other things:

1 **Avoid and Replace.** Identify as far as possible, using the information in this chapter, which toxins you think you have been exposed to/are being exposed to, and avoid them as far as possible. This includes replacing toxic versions of everyday items like perfume and toothpaste and aftershave with safer versions, as above, replacing your washing-up liquid with one by Suma (Ecoleaf) or Ecover or similar safe products, and replacing aluminium pots (and stainless-steel ones if nickel toxicity may be an issue) with safer cookware, made of materials such as cast iron, bamboo, ceramic, glass and enamel. And it involves eating organic, otherwise you are still eating biocides, hormones and antibiotics. Of course it isn't possible to avoid pollutants completely. But so far as possible, for detoxing to be successful you want to try to avoid "retoxing".

2 **Look after your nutrition,** as per the rest of this book. Toxins are far more dangerous to malnourished people than to well-nourished people. Low levels of essential minerals will give heavy metals easy access to your system, and low iodine similarly gives toxic halogens easy access. Conversely, good levels of essential minerals and vitamins will protect you. The

liver enzymes which actually do our detoxification for us (all the detox methods are just to help them along) rely heavily on vitamins and minerals as "co-factors" – vital helpers. So the golden rule here is, as in the Introduction, Put the Good Stuff In Before you try to Take the Bad Stuff Out!

3 Look after your gut, as per Chapter 2. Friendly TTCs will help you detox; unfriendly gut bugs will impede the process.

Testing For Toxins

Sadly, the NHS doesn't really test for toxicity; there are "Poisons Units" at major hospitals, but they are just looking for episodes of extreme acute poisoning. For example, if you've just bitten a mercury thermometer (some people do still have them at home), they will find mercury in your bloodstream for a couple of hours. It will be gone from the bloodstream (but not from the body) in a day or two, because the body is clever, and tries to get toxins "out of the way". But there is no "out of the way" in the body, just as we now know that there is no "away" on the planet where we can throw our rubbish. So the toxins will land up in our fat, and in organs such as the liver, kidneys, bones and brain. We can't go around doing biopsies of the liver etc. to look for toxic substances, but it would be very easy to biopsy fat; just as easy as taking blood – remember fat is liquid in the body. This would show up a lot of lipophilic (fat-soluble) toxins like pesticides, VOCs like dry-cleaning solvents and so on, if they looked for them. That's where they are hiding; in the fat, not in the blood.

Outside of the NHS, there are various ways of looking for toxins. Great Plains Laboratory do urine tests that look for the metabolites of numerous toxins; metabolites are the substances that your body has turned the toxins into (in an attempt at detoxification). Their tests are available through Biolab in London. Similarly there is the Melisa test for heavy metals, that looks at how your white blood cells react to those metals; technically it is looking for sensitivity rather than toxicity, but it's still a useful indicator. Biolab does a urine test for fluoride levels too; I find it sky-high in people from the West Midlands (and their iodine levels concomitantly low). To do a test at Biolab you need a referral from a qualified practitioner, but it doesn't have to be a doctor – it can be a nutritional therapist registered with BANT (see the Resources section).

Through Lifecode Gx, you can do a genetic test to find out what your inherent capacity for detoxification is. If your detox enzymes work well, you need to worry less about toxicity than if the test shows your detox capacity is poor, although if it is poor there is masses you can do nutritionally to boost it, and the test results will tell you what you need to do to compensate for your particular genetic "glitches". Although you can order this test on your own, you will need a qualified practitioner to interpret the results for you; Lifecode Gx should be able to recommend someone in your area, or see the Resources section.

How To Detox – The Seven Major Methods

The seven main methods I use are:

🌿 Saunas

🌿 Vegetable juicing

🌿 Epsom salts baths

🌿 Colonic hydrotherapy/irrigation

🌿 Specific supplements

🌿 High-dose Vitamin C

🌿 Sprouting

Saunas

Sweating is the best way to eliminate toxins, and is particularly useful to get rid of fat-soluble toxins, because there is a layer of fatty tissue just under the skin. Some of the people who suffer most from their encounters with chemical pollutants are precisely those who do not sweat much. Anything that encourages sweating is good, particularly exercise and saunas. It is very important to wipe off the sweat every few minutes, otherwise the toxins released from the tissues onto the skin will simply be reabsorbed by the skin. Just five or ten minutes in the sauna is sufficient – longer can be counterproductive – ideally three times per week for a few months. Your local leisure centre should have a sauna. It has to be the sauna, not the steam room, because the sweat has to be able to evaporate.

Always take a couple of large towels into the sauna with you, one to sit on and one to regularly mop up the sweat. After the sauna, put them in the laundry. Then shower. Straight after the sauna, you need to replace not only the water, but also the major minerals that will have been lost in the sweat. So take an electrolyte (mineral) solution such as "E-lyte" electrolyte concentrate by BodyBio, which replaces not only the sodium and chloride but also the potassium and magnesium, and which is, at time of writing, junk-free.

For people who cannot use an ordinary sauna, such as those with severe CFS/ME, those who have had lymph nodes removed as part of surgical treatment for breast cancer, and those who just cannot tolerate intense heat, there is a good alternative, called the Far InfraRed sauna. There are various versions of the Far InfraRed sauna, and they can be expensive, so see if there is an option to rent for a while before you buy. A UK company with a lot of experience in this field is called Get Fitt.

Vegetable juicing

This means making your own raw, organic, green vegetable juice at home. Get a good size, good-quality juicer (details below), and use only organically grown vegetables, otherwise you are juicing pesticide residues, which defeats the object. Examples of vegetables to use include:

- Celery

- Cucumber

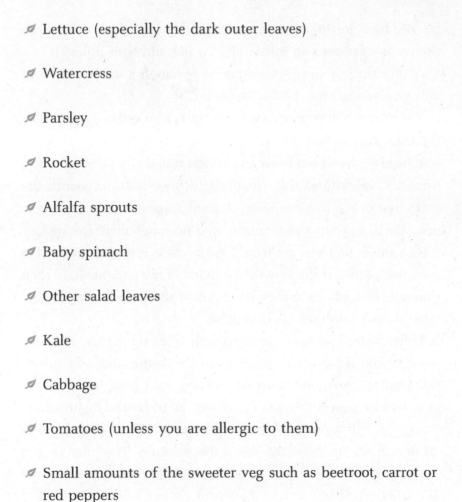

- Lettuce (especially the dark outer leaves)

- Watercress

- Parsley

- Rocket

- Alfalfa sprouts

- Baby spinach

- Other salad leaves

- Kale

- Cabbage

- Tomatoes (unless you are allergic to them)

- Small amounts of the sweeter veg such as beetroot, carrot or red peppers

You will initially want to get a balance between the sweet ones such as carrot and beetroot, and the dark green leaves. As you get used to it, gradually use more of the latter and less of the former, ideally until the juice is only green ingredients. Your taste buds will change!

Experiment with different combinations, and buy a good book

on vegetable juicing from a health-food shop, but do make sure the recipes are for **veg** juice only. Do not add fruit unless it is a very thin sliver of apple or a squeeze of lemon juice. Juicing fruit will give you too much of a "sugar hit".

The purpose of vegetable juicing is to cleanse the gut and thus the liver, to give the liver maximum capacity to do its detox work. Juicing also provides a fresh and concentrated source of vitamins, minerals and natural antioxidants, which we need to quench the toxic free radicals in our body. A good supply of antioxidants is essential to any detox programme, and no supplement can replace the goodness that you get from freshly made vegetable juice. It is hard work but it really is worth it; many of my patients have seen dramatic benefits once they have put in the work to build vegetable juicing into their daily routine.

If the vegetables have come straight from the fridge, you may need to add a little hot water from the kettle and mix before drinking. It is not good to drink anything stone cold. In the winter you can take simply take the veg out of the fridge the night before. Start with half a pint and build up to a pint. Don't swig it down all in one go; sip it gently over a few minutes. The juice should not, ideally, be made hours in advance, or it will lose much of its antioxidant power.

Which juicer to get? You need a masticating juicer, not a centrifugal one. The centrifugal ones are designed for fruit, and chunky veg such as carrots, whereas you need one that will extract maximum juice from green leaves, i.e. a masticating juicer. Check out Omega Vert and the Omega Horizontal range and VitalMax. Many of my patients have found "UK Juicers" to be helpful; they will talk you through the options: tel 01904 757070. It can be helpful to watch a video of how to set it up and use it – there are quite a few on YouTube.

A juicer is not the same as a blender. Blenders such as the NutriBullet make veg smoothies, not veg juice. Smoothies still have all the raw veg fibre in, which is ok for some people's guts but not for others, and you can get the raw fibre by simply eating a salad anyway. A smoothie-maker is just pre-chewing your salad very small for you, whereas a juicer extracts far more of the beneficial phyto-nutrients from the green leaves, so is more valuable for nutrition and detox. You can put the leftover dry pulp on the compost heap.

Epsom salts baths

This method is tried and tested, being many hundreds of years old, and is more valuable than ever in today's stressed and polluted world. Epsom salts are magnesium sulphate, and if you put ½ lb to 1lb (approx. 250–500g) of Epsom salts into the bath every night or every other night for a few months, and lie in it for 20–30 minutes, you will absorb a substantial amount of magnesium sulphate through the skin.

Almost all of us are magnesium deficient, for reasons to do with diet, stress and pollution, and it is in fact easier to absorb magnesium through the skin than it is orally. Magnesium, as we have seen, is vital for relaxation of muscles, maintenance of normal blood sugar, bone structure and at least one hundred crucial enzyme reactions within the body. But it also helps push toxic metals out of the body. The sulphate, which is the other component of Epsom salts, is extremely helpful too, as it supports some of the liver's detoxification pathways. Some people who are sulphate-sensitive may not be able to take it, but this is quite unusual.

Please note: Do NOT use soap or shampoo or any other products in an Epsom salts bath. The soap may combine with the Epsom salts and create scum. Shower first if you need to, but the point of the Epsom salts bath is to soak and absorb the magnesium sulphate – not to wash. Turn the lights down, light a candle, burn some essential oil of lavender or rose or whatever you like, play some music and enjoy!

An Epsom salts bath before bed is very relaxing and helps sleep, and Professor Rosemary Waring of Birmingham University found it to be particularly useful for autistic children, for reasons to do with their specific abnormalities of sulphate metabolism[237] as well as their need for the calming effects of magnesium.

Colonic hydrotherapy/irrigation

The main organ of detoxification is the liver. You cannot wash out your liver but you can wash out your colon, and there is an active circulation of blood from the colon to the liver, so this is the next best thing; the idea is to make the blood supply that reaches the liver from the colon as pure as possible, minimising the amount the liver has to detox, thereby maximising its capacity to detox whatever remains.

The colon is a major organ of elimination, and many toxins can be eliminated directly via the gut. Furthermore, colonic hydrotherapy tones up the muscle of the bowel wall and makes it work more efficiently, as well as removing the "plaque" that may have accumulated on the lining over decades of sub-optimal bowel function. But it does not flush out the good bacteria, any more than watering your garden washes away the plants; the significant gut bacteria are embedded in the lining of your colon, not floating around loose!

It only makes sense to start colonic hydrotherapy once you have "cleaned up" your diet, as described in this book. An improvement in what goes into your system at the top end means you'll get much more value out of clearing out the lower end! You cannot use colonic hydrotherapy as a substitute for eating good food, nor is it a tool for weight loss. Nor should you do it repeatedly; after the first three or four sessions, it should be an occasional treatment, maybe three or four times a year.

If you are unfamiliar with colonic hydrotherapy it may seem like a strange idea, but most people find it immensely helpful and not at all unpleasant. However, there are certain people for whom it is not suitable, including anyone under 18, or anyone with Inflammatory Bowel Disease (Ulcerative Colitis or Crohn's Disease). To ensure that you find a fully qualified practitioner, go via ARCH, the Association and Register of Colon Hydrotherapists – www.colonic-association.org – and speak to the practitioner before booking; it is an unusual and intimate procedure, and it is vital that you feel comfortable with the practitioner before you begin.

Specific supplements

In addition to the above four methods, which are general to the process of detoxification, there are specific supplements that are almost always helpful, such as Vitamin C, the B vitamins (to help the methylation pathways which are crucial to detoxification), zinc and magnesium (to help defend against toxic metals), Phosphatidyl Choline (PC) to help remove fat-soluble toxins, and Glutathione for many of the liver's detox pathways. Glutathione can be taken as a supplement, but is also present in most animal proteins. We vary in our capacity to make Glutathione, and the detoxification genetics test from Lifecode Gx (page 296) can tell you how well your body synthesises it, therefore whether a supplement would be helpful.

For getting rid of aluminium, silica is excellent. For getting rid of cadmium, you need zinc, Vitamin C and PC, but cadmium is very slow to go, and you may need specialist help with this, including intravenous treatment, if you were at some point in your life a smoker. For excess copper (from the pill or the coil), zinc is helpful, and for mercury toxicity there are many useful nutrients, including selenium, sulphur, iodine, zinc, Vitamin C, PC, Chlorella and cilantro. Re cilantro (coriander), it is vital that it be organically grown. This is because cilantro is as good at picking up toxic metals from the soil as it is at picking them up from our bodies, so it is only safe and effective if it has grown in uncontaminated (i.e. organic) soil. For getting rid of lead, I would use zinc, Vitamin C, PC and calcium, having checked the magnesium level first. But one can never get all the lead out, I suspect, as it hides in the bones. For nickel detox one needs (again) zinc and Vitamin C, and also the amino acid methionine. To get rid of fluoride, chlorine, bromine or bromide, one needs to use a supplement that has a combination of iodine and iodide, such as Iodoral, Iodizyme or Lugol's Iodine.

And for helping the liver with clearing virtually any toxin, milk-thistle is a very useful herb[238] – see Graham's case history on page 263.

Using Vitamin C as a medicine for detox

For getting rid of heavy metals, Vitamin C is invaluable, but to be effective one needs to use it as a medicine rather than a supplement, i.e. at higher doses than you need for regular nutritional maintenance. One needs to build up the daily dose gradually and systematically, to find one's individual "bowel tolerance", i.e. how much you can take before it (harmlessly) gives you the runs. This dose varies greatly between people; a few people can only take a gram a day, in divided doses, but people with a life-long tendency to constipation are often fine on 6 or even 10 grams daily; it's a great treatment for constipation and for gut dysbiosis generally. And, like iodine, it's a powerful antibacterial. The more one can spread out the Vitamin C doses over the day, the more one can take; it is water-soluble, so it doesn't last long.

Here's how to do it:

Get a good quality Vitamin C in the form of ascorbate, not ascorbic acid. Ascorbic acid may be cheaper, but it can be rough on the stomach. In the ascorbate form, Vitamin C is "buffered" by being combined with a mineral such as magnesium or potassium. So you are looking for magnesium ascorbate or potassium ascorbate powder. DON'T ever get an effervescent, coloured, flavoured variety; you don't want the artificial additives in there. Just pure ascorbate.

Why powder, not capsules? Because the large doses of Vitamin C you need for detox purposes (as opposed to the much lower dosage for regular nutritional maintenance) would require you to swallow too many capsules, overloading your digestive system with methyl cellulose (the stuff most capsules are made of).

Dissolve the Vitamin C powder in water or vegetable juice or, last choice, *very* diluted fruit juice. Vegetable juice is best (home-made of course). Water is fine if you are ok with the taste of the Vitamin C – most people don't mind it. Fruit juice is bad news because it gives you a sugar hit, so if you really can't take your Vitamin C powder any other way, at least dilute the fruit juice 1:2 with water.

This is how to build up the amount, over a six-day period:

(A teaspoon is 4–5 g)
Day 1: 1 g at breakfast
Day 2: 1 g at breakfast
        1 g at dinner
Day 3: 1 g at breakfast
        1 g at lunch
        1 g at dinner
Day 4: 2 g at breakfast
        1 g at lunch
        1 g at dinner
Day 5: 2 g at breakfast
        1 g at lunch
        2 g at dinner
Day 6 and thereafter: 2 g at each meal

Most people won't need to go any higher than this. If at any point in this increasing schedule you get "the runs", you may have exceeded your "bowel tolerance" for Vitamin C. So, drop down to the previous day's dose, and stick to it; that is your personal maximum. In practice, I find it's very rare for bowel tolerance to be as low as 6 g per day, so long as the doses are spread out. If you forget the lunchtime dose, DON'T double up at dinner. If you forgot, you forgot. Let it go. Vitamin C is water-soluble, so the body pees out what it can't use up within a matter of hours. So you need it frequently, but there is probably no advantage to taking more than 2 g at once, in most situations.

Vitamin C at these (relatively) high doses is useful for combating unfriendly bacteria/fungal organisms in the gut, as well as for shifting heavy metals and other toxins safely out of the body. And of course it helps the immune system to keep infections at bay.

You don't need to do this for more than a few months. After that you can drop down to ½ g at breakfast and ½ g at dinner, and that means you can use 500 mg (½ g) capsules. If you feel run down, or people around you are full of coughs and colds, you can increase it again as needed, to support your immune defences.

For more information about Vitamin C, you can do no better than check out the work of Nobel prize-winning scientist Linus Pauling.

Sprouting

Detoxification can occasionally drain the good minerals out of your system as well as the toxic heavy metals. The best way to prevent this, in addition to taking the necessary supplements, is to sprout your own seeds and beans. This is very easy, and is described in the Spring chapter.

Sprouting is a good practice for life, not just for the period of detox. It is like having a tiny, organic, instant allotment in your kitchen. Immensely beneficial nutritionally, even if you're not detoxing.

Electro-Magnetic Radiation

Well, this whole chapter has only been about CHEMICAL toxicity. There is another equally hazardous source of environmental pollution and illness, namely ELECTRO-MAGNETIC RADIATION (EMR; see page 167), from our mobile phones, mobile phone masts, wifi, and more. There hasn't been space to explore it here – it will have to go in another book – but as with chemical pollution, there are plenty of ways to protect yourself. Some useful websites are listed in the resources section. Meanwhile, many doctors in the UK and around the world are extremely worried not only about existing levels of EMR, but even more about the imminent arrival of 5G, which has been banned by some sensible European cities, and which will have damaging effects on all parts of our bodies, and particularly our brains. Concerned doctors have formed an organisation called PHIRE – Physicians' Health Initiative for Radiation and Environment (www.phiremedical.org).

It's very important not to sink into despair about all this; there is plenty we can and must do about it, both individually and together. Of course it is hard to know all this stuff; I'd rather not know, in a way! But it is better to light one candle than to curse the darkness.

CONCLUSION

The reason I've written this book is to enable you to become healthy, energetic and clear-headed. Partly so you can enjoy life more, but also so you can be well enough to play your part, however small, in helping to save our one and only precious planet. Our health and that of the planet are inextricably linked. Having cleaned up our bodies, we need to clean up our act, clean up our mother, the Earth. So that there is a safe and healthy future for all our children.

APPENDIX

....

A Rough Guide to Some Major Nutrients

This book has referred frequently to various vitamins and minerals, especially under "pre-conception nutrition" in Chapter 5, but hasn't defined them, or set them in the context of all the other sorts of nutrients we also need. There isn't space here for a systematic survey of all the vitamins and minerals – that will have to wait for another book. So I will just offer simple definitions of vitamins and minerals, and then rather more information about the other five major groups of nutrients that haven't featured so prominently in the book.

The seven main categories of nutrients are:

- Minerals

- Vitamins

- Proteins

- Carbohydrates

🌿 Fats

🌿 Fibre

🌿 Water

Perhaps we should add two more categories: Phytonutrients (all the goodies we get from plants that are neither minerals nor vitamins) and friendly bacteria, the TTCs I have referred to throughout the book. But for now, we'll stick to the generally recognised seven types.

Minerals

Minerals are elements (as opposed to compound substances) that we need in our bodies. Some we require in large amounts, like sodium, potassium, calcium and magnesium, and others in much smaller amounts, like iron, zinc, iodine, sulphur, silicon, selenium, chromium, manganese, copper, molybdenum, cobalt, boron and vanadium. Whether we get enough minerals depends on whether the soil in which our food was grown has been depleted by intensive farming, and on whether these good minerals are having to compete with toxic metals in our environment, and on whether our stomach is producing enough acid to enable us to absorb the minerals. Sadly, people on protein-pump inhibitor drugs like Omeprazole will not be producing sufficient stomach acid to absorb all their minerals. Taking liquid mineral supplements as opposed to capsules/tablets may help a little with this problem.

Vitamins

Vitamins are compounds that are essential, in tiny amounts, for our bodies to work, but that we cannot synthesise in our cells, so we have to take them in with our food. Vitamin C and the B vitamin group are water-soluble – we need some every day, because we can't store them; we pee out any spare within a few hours. By contrast, vitamins A, D, E and K are fat-soluble, so they do hang around in the body. This means that you can build up a supply and then manage without for a while. For example, if you are lucky enough to be sunbathing from May to September, you'll build up enough Vitamin D to see you through to December. On the other hand, because we store these vitamins, it is possible to overdose; hence the need for testing from time to time.

Proteins

From the Greek "I am first", protein is what we are mostly made of, apart from water. Our muscles are more or less pure protein. Our bones, interestingly, are made of protein as well as minerals. Our connective tissue (ligaments, tendons and more) is largely protein. The enzymes that catalyse (facilitate and speed up) all the thousands of biochemical reactions in the body are proteins. Our nerve cells are made of protein, and so is our heart. The antibodies of our immune system are also proteins.

Proteins are large molecules composed of many much smaller molecules called amino acids, strung together; there are more than 20. We need to eat some protein most days either from animal food (meat, fish, eggs, cheese, yogurt) or from vegan sources such as nuts, seeds, peas, beans, lentils and so on. When these latter are judiciously combined with whole grains, vegans can get their full complement of amino acids – just.

When we eat protein foods, our digestive enzymes break them down (if all is working well) into their constituent amino acids. We then absorb these, and then rearrange them into the order pre-determined by our genes, which are our blueprints. That's what your DNA is doing all day when it's not dividing; arranging amino acids in the correct order to make the protein of your skin, your eyes, your spleen and so on. Each of them is different from each other, and from someone else's skin, eyes and spleen. And very different from the original protein you ate. It is the order of the amino acids that decides the appearance and function of all living tissues. That's why you can eat beef without looking like a cow, or eat lentils without looking like a lentil. We rearrange.

You don't need protein supplements. You don't need protein shakes or protein bars, however hard you work out at the gym. You just need some protein food. Protein drinks are junk. Check the ingredients list. Our hunter-gatherer ancestors did quite a workout and managed without them. EAT your protein – the only people who need to DRINK their protein are babies.

Carbohydrates

Carbohydrates, found in grains and tubers and root veg and bananas, are an energy source – our main fuel, although not the only one. Rice, sweetcorn, oats, bread, pasta and potatoes are the commonest carbohydrate foods in the UK. Children, I believe, do need some carbohydrates every day, for energy. Some adults can manage without for quite a while; we can break down fat, and even protein if necessary, to make energy. This is what we do if fasting or in conditions of starvation. But kids need to keep their protein for growing; they don't want to have to break it down for energy, so they need their carbs for that purpose.

Carbohydrates are large molecules (although not nearly as large as proteins) composed of smaller molecules which are sugars. There are three main single sugars, or monosaccharides: glucose, fructose and galactose. They combine to make double sugars, or disaccharides. The double sugars are sucrose (table sugar, composed of glucose + fructose), lactose (milk sugar, composed of glucose + galactose) and maltose (composed of two glucose molecules).

Starch – pure carbohydrate – is made up of many of these sugar molecules strung together, so is called a polysaccharide. When our digestive enzymes break carbohydrates down, they first break them into disaccharides, and then other enzymes break the disaccharides down into monosaccharides, which are absorbed into the bloodstream. As we've seen, the slower this last process happens the better, in terms of blood sugar stability. This leads onto the debate about whole, "brown" carbohydrates versus refined, "white" carbohydrates.

Whole grains have a white, starchy centre, which is pure polysaccharide, and a brown outer husk which contains fibre, B vitamins and the mineral chromium. Now that's handy; the fibre nicely slows down the digestion of the starchy middle bit, so the blood sugar level doesn't rise too quickly (which would trigger an insulin rush). And the B vitamins, especially vitamin B1 (thiamine) assist with sugar metabolism later on, in the cells. And the chromium helps insulin to do its job properly,[239] thus regulating blood sugar levels. So the whole grain is a useful combined package. Furthermore, inside the "germ" in the middle of the grain is the germ oil, e.g. wheat germ oil, which is a rich natural source of Vitamin E.

When whole grains are processed into white grains like white rice, or white wheat to make white flour, white bread and white pasta, all these good bits are removed. Trashed. So we are left with pure starch, pure polysaccharide: refined carbohydrate. When we eat it, it gets broken down to sugar so fast that it's almost as bad as eating sugar itself.

So why do they do it? Commercial reasons. Whole grains don't store so well; they are "alive", so they can go off. White flour is a dead substance; lasts for ever on the supermarket shelves. And it's addictive; it doesn't really fill you up in a satisfying way, but gives you an empty sugar rush, and creates the desire for more and more of the same. Very profitable. Constipating, too.

Did I say they trash the good bits? Actually, they don't. They remove them, but then sell them back to us separately as wheat germ oil and bran. Cheeky, I call it. Rice is the staple food in east Asia. When it began to be processed and refined in the 19th century, and turned into white rice, people began to die of Beriberi. That's the disease that results from total absence of Vitamin B1, thiamine. Most people were poor and didn't have enough animal food to provide an alternative source of Vitamin B1; they relied on rice. And they died.

So whole grains are good for you, right? Well, that was the belief in the "health food movement" from the 1970s onwards, and of the macrobiotic people for much longer, for all the reasons given above. But now there is a school of thought that says they are BAD for you! Some people point out that they contain phytates, which can prevent essential minerals (especially iron, calcium and zinc) from being absorbed in the gut.[240,241] This is true, but there are plenty of traditional methods to reduce the phytate content of grains, such as soaking, thorough cooking, sprouting (see Spring chapter) and fermentation.[242] Boil your muesli and turn it into porridge; raw grains are not good for the gut.

Others point out that whole grains, along with legumes (peas/beans/lentils), also contain lectins, some of which are toxic.[243] Still others make the evolutionary argument that we've only been eating grains (and legumes/pulses, and dairy) since the agricultural revolution, max 10,000 years ago. And that is actually very recent in terms of our physiological evolution; a mere blip compared with millions of years as hunter-gatherers living on green plants, meat and fish.

There are books with titles like "No Grain, No Pain" and "Grain Brain". These authors are not advocating refined grains as opposed to whole grains. They're advocating no grains at all. It's part of the "Paleo" (Stone Age) diet approach. So what to do?

Suck it and see. Everyone's different. Everything in moderation. I keep waiting for the Age of Reason to dawn in the nutritional world, but we still seem to be in the Age of Extremes. Some whole grains are fine for some people, some of the time. That's my simple, not-so-radical, unfashionable view.

But what about **GLUTEN**? Gluten is a protein (really a group of proteins) found in some grains but not in others. (Yes, grains are basically a carbohydrate food, but they contain some protein as well.) Here's a list:

- **Gluten-containing grains:** wheat, spelt (wild wheat), rye, barley and most oats

- **Gluten-free grains:** rice, maize (sweetcorn), buckwheat, quinoa, millet and some obscure ones like amaranth, sorghum and teff, and gluten-free oats

Is gluten a problem? For some people yes, for others no. In people with full-blown coeliac disease, gluten damages the lining of their small intestine to the point where it becomes unable to absorb essential nutrients, especially the vital Vitamin B12.

Testing for coeliac disease and gluten sensitivity

Hospital doctors test for coeliac disease by doing an endoscopy (tube down into the gut) and taking a biopsy of the jejunum (part of the small intestine). If they see damage to the villi (the tiny folds of the gut lining which facilitate absorption by increasing surface area) they will make a diagnosis of coeliac disease. But there is a whole spectrum of gluten sensitivity from none at all to full-on coeliac disease. The people in the middle (gluten-sensitive, but not coeliac) are only just starting to be recognised by the medical profession at large.

A problem with this standard approach to testing and diagnosis, apart from its invasiveness, is that it only yields a positive result if the person has been eating lots of gluten in the weeks leading up to the test. But if you suspect you have gluten sensitivity/coeliac disease, and therefore have been conscientiously avoiding gluten, the test will be negative. That

---

does not necessarily mean that gluten is not problematic for you, it just means that during the weeks of avoiding it, the villi of the cells lining your small intestine have had a chance to recover and regrow.

Several of my patients who have been avoiding gluten for some time and have started feeling much better as a result (gut working better, energy and mood improved) have been told that they need to eat several slices of bread daily for 6 weeks, and then have the biopsy. Some of them get quite ill doing this, which only confirms that they are sensitive to gluten (or possibly just wheat – see below), and choose to go back to the gluten-free diet that has been working well for them, and not have the test. There is also a blood test for gluten-sensitivity, which looks for antibodies which your body may be making against gluten. This also will only yield a positive result if you have been eating gluten-containing foods recently, but it is far less invasive.

It is possible to do a version of the "Elimination and Reintroduction" protocol for gluten sensitivity, which takes account of the fact that some people may react badly to wheat but not to the other gluten grains. What you do is to cut out ALL the gluten-contaning grains (see list opposite) for 2 weeks, and then reintroduce all five of them gradually, leaving a 48-hour gap between reintroductions because the grains can take that long to produce symptoms. The order of reintroduction is important; you start with the one least likely to cause a problem, and end with the most likely culprit. So the order is, after a fortnight of strictly no gluten at all:

Day 1 – barley

Day 3 – ordinary oats

Day 5 – rye

Day 7 – spelt

Day 9 – wheat (as pasta)

Day 11 – wheat as bread (just in case you are reacting to the
   yeast, not the wheat)

Observe and record any symptoms, mental/emotional as well as physical, and you should have your answer. If any grain gives you symptoms, wait until those symptoms have completely cleared before proceeding to introduce the other grains. The point of the exercise is to see whether any or all of these grains are a problem for you; some people will react to all of them, in which case gluten is indeed the problem. But plenty of people find they are fine with all these grains except for wheat. This is important, because it means they do NOT need to miss out on rye, barley, oats etc. – becoming wheat-free is simpler and less restrictive than being fully gluten-free.

If you get a bad reaction to the first three grains on the list, then you are indeed gluten-sensitive, and there is no point in proceeding to introduce spelt and wheat, because they are even higher in gluten and will probably give you a stronger reaction. Some people are ok with spelt (the original form of wheat before it was selectively bred) and not with wheat; others can't take either. Suck it and see.

Coeliac disease itself has long been recognised, and was initially called "Failure to Thrive" in babies, when its cause wasn't understood. But it's the not-quite-coeliac gluten-sensitivity that has become far commoner than it used to be. Some people get bloating, diarrhoea or constipation from food containing the gluten grains, and others develop psychiatric or neurological symptoms,[244] with or even without the gastro-intestinal effects. Some people get skin reactions. Excluding gluten (and also casein, the main protein in dairy products) from the diet does seem to lead to particular improvements in children with autism;[245] I have noticed especially some improvement in eye contact and social interaction within 2–4 months.

Why has gluten sensitivity become so common? It may be partly because our bread now contains much more gluten than the bread of 100 years ago; wheat has been bred to contain more gluten. But gluten sensitivity may also be increasing for the same reason that other food intolerances are on the increase: Toxicant-Induced Loss of Tolerance, or TILT (see page 93). And I'm sure there are other reasons yet to be discovered.

But gluten is certainly not the only problem with modern bread; all sorts of additives are added to flour which don't need to be declared on the label. And if you read what IS on the label of most commerically produced bread, it's quite disturbing. Unfortunately, most commercially produced gluten-free breads are every bit as bad. If you find you do have to be gluten-free, you don't need to buy this junk bread. You can cook the gluten-free grains, and you can cook noodles or pasta made from them; most health-food shops stock buckwheat pasta, rice pasta, black rice noodles and so on which are quick and easy to cook, and not full of additives. And you can learn to bake your own gluten-free bread.

Finally, we've been talking about grains, but what about potatoes, sweet potatoes, pumpkins, yams, butternut squash, turnips, swedes, carrots and so on? These are all carbohydrate foods, but we've been eating them, or root veg like them, for far, far longer than the grains (see page 48). So they are not problematic for the vast majority of people. It is best to eat them with their skins on (assuming they're organic) where the skin is edible, for maximum fibre to balance the polysaccharide content.

Fats

This section should really be called "Fats and Oils". Fats are solid at room temperature, oils are liquid at room temperature. Our bodies, at around 37 degrees centigrade, are much warmer than the average room, so all the fat in our bodies is in liquid form; effectively, it is oil.

When I was at medical school we were taught that the sole purposes of fat were insulation, protective padding and as a concentrated energy reserve. Certainly fat has all these functions, but we now know it has many more besides. Fat cells, or adipocytes, are active participants in metabolism and in the regulation of our immune system, and fats are also essential components of our cell membranes.

The collective term for fats, oils and related substances is **lipids**. One of the most important lipids is the vital but much-maligned **cholesterol**. We make it in our liver, and turn it into many different substances, including bile for our digestion, Vitamin D (with the help of sunlight on the skin), the hormones cortisol and aldosterone and the sex hormones oestrogen, progesterone and testosterone. Our brains and bodies need it; we can't live without it.

Debate is raging about good fats and bad fats, saturated/unsaturated fats, hydrogenated fats and trans fats. Without going into detailed biochemistry of the molecular structures of these different types of fat, what follows contains some simple take-home messages about the nature of these fats, which to eat and which to avoid.

Saturated fats tend to be solid at room temperature, whereas **unsaturated** ones are liquid, so they are in fact oils. Most animal fats are saturated, and most vegetable oils are unsaturated. There are exceptions, such as coconut oil, a saturated fat that is solid on a winter's day but liquid on a hot summer's day.

For over 40 years there was a myth that saturated fats were bad for us. But much of our own body fat is saturated – it's animal fat, because we are animals. Saturated fat is very bad for rabbits, because they are herbivores. But it's ok for us, in moderation. It's not essential, though, because we can make it for ourselves.

Unsaturated fats – basically vegetable oils – are good for us, but ONLY if they're produced in the time-honoured way, by physically crushing the olive, or the sunflower seed, or the hemp seed or the sesame seed, or whatever. This is the cold-pressing method, and it preserves the oil in its safe form. These oils need to be kept in dark glass bottles, in the fridge, and protected from air, light and heat. They are fragile. Don't cook with them; use them cold and raw on salads.

What's not ok at all are oils that have been produced from the seed/nut/soya bean etc by chemical extraction, heat treatment and other industrial processes. This is the refined oil that you see in plastic bottles in supermarkets. It looks like wee and it's not fit for human consumption.

Trans fats

When a vegetable oil is heated to a high temperature (e.g. chip-frying temperature) it may flip into the "trans" form, which has the effect of straightening out the molecule and making it rigid, so it obstructs cell membranes and does all sorts of damage in the body, most notably increasing the risk of heart disease.[246] Trans fats are unnatural and are now, at last, being recognised as dangerous, and are slowly being removed from a vast number of processed and packaged foods. But they're not gone yet.

Unsaturated fats are delicate, and all sorts of commercial food-processing as well as the high temperatures used in chip frying change them chemically in many ways; the possible production of toxic trans fats is just one of the risks.[247,248,249,250,251] However, when it comes to saturated fats such as lard or dripping or lamb fat or chicken fat or duck fat or butter or ghee or coconut oil, you can safely cook with them without doing any damage. They don't change their molecular structure when heated (unless you BBQ them to the point of charred blackness). They are stable.

This makes sense; the animal fat in our own bodies is at 37 degrees centigrade, and that's fine. But vegetable oil comes from plants, and most plants will **not** be fine if you heat them to 37 degrees; they'll shrivel up.

Hydrogenated fats

So much for trans fats – bad. What about hydrogenated fats? What does that mean? Well, what margarine manufacturers have done is to take a vegetable oil, such as sunflower oil, which is naturally unsaturated, and saturate it with hydrogen atoms in the factory (at high temperatures, using the toxic metal nickel as a catalyst). Why on earth would they do that? If we want a solid, saturated fat to spread on our bread, we've got butter! They have artificially saturated a vegetable **oil** with hydrogen atoms – in other words, **hydrogen-ated** it – in order to make it into a synthetic vegetable **fat** – solid like butter, looking like butter, but tasting nothing like butter however hard they try. Margarine is unnatural, toxic and pointless. But it has proven extremely profitable; the manufacturers seized on some very dodgy research to frighten us out of our wits about butter, and convince us that their artificial chemical substitute was safer. The reverse is the case. Margarine is made **from** vegetable oil, but it is so processed that it no longer bears any resemblance to vegetable oil. If it was vegetable **oil**, it would be sloshing around in the tub, spilling out. I might grease a squeaky door hinge with marg, but I wouldn't eat it.

Cooking with olive oil

Do we have to use olive oil only raw, or can we also cook with it? Opinion is divided. My take on it is that people in the Mediterranean countries have been using olive oil both cooked and raw for centuries. But please note, they cook with it at fairly low temperatures; they most certainly do not fry chips in it! So I reckon we are safe to sauté veg or cook an omelette in it (and Professor Tim Spector agrees.)[252] But for a longer, hotter, stir-fried meal I would use coconut oil instead – or, yes, animal fat. You don't have to buy the animal fat though; just keep the fat that drains off the chicken or whatever meat you are cooking. It will keep for at least a week in the fridge. Obviously vegetarians and vegans won't do this, but vegans can use coconut oil, and vegetarians can use coconut oil or butter or ghee.

Essential Fatty Acids

Some Poly-Unsaturated Fatty Acids (PUFAs) are essential constituents of our bodies and brains, particularly our cell membranes. They also have a vital role in both fighting inflammation and, where necessary for our self-defence, promoting it. They are the "parent molecules" for such vital substances as prostaglandins, prostacyclins, thromboxanes and leukotrienes, all of which we can make from them, if we have sufficient zinc, magnesium, Vitamin C and the B vitamins. (And we also need Vitamin E to keep all the fatty acids in our body in the healthy, non-oxidised state. So you see how hard it is in reality to disentangle one nutrient from another; they all need each other, so we need all of them.)

These fatty acids are as essential as vitamins and minerals, so are known as Essential Fatty Acids, or **EFAs**. We cannot make them for ourselves, so we have to eat them. You will have heard about **Omega 3** and **Omega 6** essential fatty acids. Omega 3 EFAs, such as EPA and DHA, are found in oily fish. They are essential for brain function, and as natural anti-inflammatories, and are excellent at stopping the blood from clotting when it shouldn't. The Inuit people of the Arctic live on fish, and while they stick to their traditional diet they do not get heart attacks. Vegetarians, who don't eat fish, can get certain omega 3 EFAs from walnut oil or flaxseed oil, but my experience of testing over many years suggests that they don't convert very well to EPA and DHA, which are the ones the brain needs most.

Omega 6 EFAs are found in a wide variety of seeds, nuts, grains, greens and plant foods generally. They also occur in meat, in the form of arachidonic acid, but the plant versions are better. They are most concentrated in cold-pressed vegetable oils (as on page 323, above) and in evening primrose oil, blackcurrant oil and borage (starflower) oil. They are good anti-inflammatories, and vital for the health of the skin, brain, circulation, immune system, reproductive system and more.

There are other "Omega-numbered" fatty acids, such as oleic acid in olive oil, which is omega 9, and sea buckthorn oil, omega 7, which is useful along with Vitamin E oil for post-menopausal vulval dryness. But omegas 3 and 6 are the main ones we need for our normal biochemistry.

Because EFAs haven't been known about and understood for as long as vitamins and minerals, we don't have a neat list of deficiency diseases caused by their absence. What we do have is a few decades of clinical experience. Here are some of the problems that I and my colleagues (in the British Society for Ecological Medicine) have seen when people are low in the EFAs:

- Excessive thirst (not due to diabetes)

- Dandruff, hair loss, eczema, dry skin, and goosebump-type pimples on the upper arms

- Varicose veins

- Poor wound healing

- Impaired mental function, especially in children

- Excess sweating

- Fatty liver (can also be due to excess sugar or alcohol intake)

- Muscle weakness and/or inflamed joints

- Heart problems

- Fertility problems

. . . and more.

We have also seen all these problems improve with supplementation of EFAs, but only as part of an overall programme of diet, exercise, vitamins and minerals as well. And all the problems listed above can have other causes too. Most serious health problems, when properly investigated, are found to have several contributory causes, not just one.

Omega 3 and omega 6 supplements

Your levels of EFAs can be tested at TDL (The Doctors' Laboratory) or Biolab in London. If you are low in omega 3s and/or omega 6s, I would take the relevant supplements, but I

---

wouldn't worry too much about the **ratio** of omega 3 to omega 6, because although everybody's talking about it, the experts can't actually agree on what the right ratio is!

For omega 3 deficiency you want a good-quality fish oil, such as those made by Nordic Naturals. They should contain DHA and EPA, and a little Vitamin E to keep them fresh, but not much else. For omega 6 deficiency I think evening primrose oil is the very best (and it's an excellent treatment for Pre-Menstrual Syndrome, along with magnesium and a B complex and Vitamin E), but blackcurrant oil and borage oil are good too. Biocare do a good Evening Primrose Oil.

There are some EFA combinations on the market that contain omegas 3, 6 and 9 together. This doesn't do you any harm, but it's not as effective as taking them separately. This is because the same enzyme delta-6-desaturase has to start working on both omega 3 and omega 6 EFAs, to convert them to their "downstream" anti-inflammatory products. It can't work on both omega 3 and omega 6 at once. It will prioritise one and neglect the other. So you'll get more mileage out of your EFA supplements if you take them separately, e.g. fish oils (omega 3) at breakfast and evening primrose (omega 6) at dinner. Or vice versa.

For women in their menstruating years, however, the best way is to take fish oils for the first half of the menstrual cycle (that's from day 1, when the period begins, to ovulation at around day 14), and to take evening primrose oil in the second half (from mid-cycle to when the next period comes, whether that's day 28 or sooner or later).

But remember, don't take fish oils indefinitely; see Dr Damien Downing's warning about this in Chapter 5 on page 162.

Fibre

This is "roughage" from all plant foods. It is essential for peristalsis, the wave-like movement of the intestines that propels food and then faeces along the gut. And, as we now know, it is vital food for our Trillions of Tiny Companions, the bacteria who live in our gastro-intestinal tract. We don't digest fibre; they digest it for us, and both we and they get the benefit.

Water

We are mostly made of it, most of us need to drink more of it, and sadly we may need to filter it, with a proper plumbed-in water filter (details in Chapter 7). That's because our tap water is chlorinated, and may also contain traces of heavy metals and residues of pesticides and herbicides that run off the fields into the reservoirs. There may even be traces of hormones peed out into the water supplies by women taking HRT and the contraceptive pill. If we leave the EU (still unclear at time of writing) then it may become legal for cows and sheep in our fields to be injected with hormones, leading to an exacerbation of this problem.

RESEARCH

···

Useful books, organisations, laboratories, websites and films

Books:

- *Nutritional Medicine* by Dr Stephen Davies and Dr Alan Stewart (Pan Books, 1987)
- *Environmental Medicine in Clinical Practice* by Anthony, Birtwistle, Eaton and Maberly (the best one for your GP) (British Society for Allergy & Environmental Medicine, 2002)
- *The Complete Guide to Food Allergy and Intolerance* by Professor Brostoff and Linda Gamlin (Quality Health Books, 2008)
- *Biochemical Individuality* by Dr Roger Williams (McGraw-Hill, 1998)
- *Nutrition and Mental Health: a handbook*, edited by Martina Watts (Pavilion Publishing, 2008)
- *Fat Chance* by Dr Robert Lustig (Fourth Estate, 2014)
- *Prevent and Cure Diabetes* by Dr Sarah Myhill and Craig Robinson (Hammersmith Health Books, 2016)
- *Sustainable Medicine* by Dr Sarah Myhill (Hammersmith Health Books, 2015)

- *Diagnosis and Treatment of Chronic Fatigue Syndrome and Myalgic Encephalitis* by Dr Sarah Myhill (Hammersmith Health Books, 2017)
- *Not on the Label* by Felicity Lawrence (Penguin, 2004)
- *Swallow This* by Joanna Blythman (Fourth Estate, 2015)
- *The Perils of Progress* by John Ashton and Ron Laura (Zen Books, 1999)
- *Cleaning Yourself to Death* by Pat Thomas (Newleaf, 2001)
- *The Case Against Fluoride* by Dr Paul Connett (Chelsea Green Publishing, 2010)
- *Iodine* by Dr David Brownstein (Medical Alternatives Press, 2009)
- *Menace in the Mouth?* by Dr Jack Levenson (What Doctors Don't Tell You Ltd., 2000)
- *Day Light Robbery* by Dr Damien Downing (Arrow Books, 1988)
- *The Vitamin Cure for Allergies* by Dr Damien Downing (Basic Health Publications, 2011)
- *Detoxify or Die* by Dr Sherry Rogers (Prestige Pubs, 2002)
- *Aerotoxic Syndrome* by Captain John Hoyte (Pilot Press, 2014)
- *Toxic Airlines* by Captain Tristan Loraine (DFT Enterprises Ltd., 2007)
- *Asthma Epidemic* by Dr John Mansfield (Thorsons, 1997)
- *Arthritis* by Dr John Mansfield (Thorsons, 1995)
- *Chemical Exposures* by Professor Nicholas Ashford and Professor Claudia Miller (Wiley-Interscience, 1998)
- *Bestfeeding* by Mary Renfrew, Chloe Fisher and Suzanne Arms (Celestial Arts, 2004)

Organisations:

- British Society for Ecological Medicine – www.bsem.org.uk
- British Association of Nutritional Therapists – www.bant.org.uk
- Academy of Nutritional Medicine – www.aonm.org
- Institute for Optimum Nutrition – www.ion.ac.uk
- College of Naturopathic Medicine – www.naturopathy-uk.com
- Centre for Nutrition Education and Lifestyle Medicine – www.cnelm.co.uk
- National Institute of Medical Herbalists – www.nimh.org.uk
- Active Birth Centre – www.activebirthcentre.com
- La Leche League – www.laleche.org.uk
- The Healthy House – www.healthy-house.co.uk
- Greenfibres – www.greenfibres.com
- The Soil Association – www.soilassociation.org
- Mercury Madness – www.mercurymadness.org
- Fluoride Action Network – www.fluoridealert.org
- Abaca mattresses – www.abacaorganic.co.uk
- Pesticide Action Network – www.pan-uk.org
- Physicians' Health Initiative for Radiation and Environment – www.phiremedical.org

Laboratories:

- Biolab – www.biolab.co.uk
- The Doctors' Laboratory – www.tdlpathology.com

Websites:

For information on electro-magnetic hazards and how to protect yourself:

- www.powerwatch.org.uk
- www.wiredchild.org
- www.tetrawatch.net
- www.emfacts.com
- www.phiremedical.org

For information on the health hazards of frequent flying and how to protect yourself:

- www.toxicfreeairlines.com
- www.aerotoxic.org
- www.angelfleet.net

For information on reducing harmful drinking:

- www.downyourdrink.org.uk

And for information on absolutely everything (medicine, nutrition, toxicity, infection, the gut and more), you can consult Dr Sarah Myhill's vast and encyclopaedic website:

- www.drmyhill.co.uk

FILMS by Captain Tristan Loraine from "Fact Not Fiction Films" (www.factnotfictionfilms.com):

- *Everybody Flies: One Man's Journey to Make Air Travel Safe*
- *A Dark Reflection*
- *Angel without Wings*

ACKNOWLEDGEMENTS

I am deeply grateful to all my colleagues in the British Society for Ecological Medicine; I have learnt so much from these brave, pioneering doctors. I must especially thank Dr Sibyl Birtwistle, my first mentor, who introduced me to this kind of medicine back in the 1990s, Dr John McLaren-Howard, a scientific genius who remains a fount of wisdom always generously shared, and Drs Damien Downing, Sarah Myhill, Shideh Pouria and Charles Forsyth, from all of whose tremendous clinical experience and extensive medical knowledge I and my patients continue to benefit greatly. I am also indebted to Drs John Mansfield, Keith Eaton and David Freed, all sadly no longer with us, who taught me so much, in the Hippocratic spirit of passing on their medical knowledge freely to other doctors.

The researcher and lecturer Dr Rachel Nicoll has kindly shared with me her impressive and wide-ranging knowledge of the large (but largely ignored) scientific literature about environmental toxins and what they do to us. I am very grateful for her time and expertise. And I am deeply grateful to my patients, for their courage and determination to persevere with a natural form of medicine that takes so much more effort and tenacity than simply popping a pill and carrying on as usual.

Dee Passon, Captain Tristan Loraine and Dr Susan Michaelis, all courageous and knowledgeable campaigners for clean, safe air on aircraft, have shared with me their detailed knowledge about Aerotoxic Syndrome, which has been immensely helpful; thank you all.

I am very grateful to my agent, Jennifer Hewson, whose idea it was to write a book about seasonal nutrition, and whose support and encouragement have been invaluable. I am also grateful to Sally Somers, who coached me patiently through the initially daunting process of editing on the computer, and to Nicky Ross, Holly Whitaker, Emma Knight, Caitriona Horne and the whole team at Yellow Kite, who have steered me patiently through everything else involved in the publishing process. It was all new to me. Thank you.

Friends and family have given invaluable moral and practical support while I've been writing this book in the midst of running a busy clinical practice. Hilary Wainer and Alexander Massey provided a quiet weekend and space to write in their garden cabin, with all meals thrown in (not literally). I have had ongoing encouragement as well as valuable feedback from Shoshi Asheri, Suzette Clough, Vivienne Cato, Jacqui Kashyap Lichtenstern and Aleda Erskine. Aleda went so far as to keep me supplied with healthy homemade lunches throughout the last three weeks of intensive writing up, so I didn't need to break my flow by stopping to cook. (This meant I didn't have to either skip lunch or eat convenience food, either of which options would have been a contradiction of every principle in this book!) And I am very grateful for the consistent, loving support of my sister, Lynda Goodman.

Jackie Draper and Ingrid Stringer took time out of their busy lives to read the manuscript, and made invaluable corrections and suggestions, which I deeply appreciate. Any remaining errors, however, are strictly my own.

Lastly, and by no means leastly, infinite gratitude to my wonderful husband Dr Stuart Linke, for his constant love, support and solidarity, encouragement and kindly, helpful criticism. Also for his skill and patience as the unofficial "IT department" every time the computer turns into an enemy alien, which it does on a regular basis. Thank you so much.

REFERENCES

1 Brunekreef B. and Holgate S.T., 2002, 'Air Pollution and Health', *The Lancet*, vol 360, issue 9341, pp 1233–1242.

2 Kampa M. and Castanas E., 2008, 'Human Health Effects of Air Pollution', *Environmental Pollution*, vol 151, issue 2, pp 362–7.

3 Senesil G.S. et al, 1999, 'Trace element inputs into soils by anthropogenic activities and implications for human health', *Chemosphere*, vol 39, issue 2, pp 343–377.

4 Patel D. and Minajagi M., 2018, 'Prevalence of vitamin D deficiency in adult patients admitted to a psychiatric hospital', *BJPsych Bulletin*, vol 42, issue 3, pp 123–126.

5 Eaton S.B. and Konnor M., 1985, 'Paleolithic Nutrition', *New England Journal of Medicine*, vol 312, no 5, pp 283–289

6 Clemente J.C., Pehrsson E.C., Blaser M.J. et al, 2015, 'The Microbiome of uncontacted Amerindians', *Science Advances*, vol 1, no 3.

7 Kaplan H., Thompson R.C., Trumble B.C. et al, 2017, 'Coronary atherosclerosis in indigenous South American

Tsimane: a cross-sectional cohort study', *The Lancet*, vol 389, issue 10080, pp 1676–1678.

8 Harari Y.N., 2011, *Sapiens - A Brief History of Humankind*, Vintage, London.

9 Chao A. et al, 2005, 'Meat consumption and risk of colorectal cancer', *JAMA*, vol 293, issue 2, pp 172–182.

10 Larsson S.C. and Wolk A., 2012, 'Red and processed meat consumption and risk of pancreatic cancer: meta-analysis of prospective studies', *Br Jnl Cancer*, vol 106, issue 3, p 603.

11 Krajcovicova-Kudlackova M. et al, 2000, 'Correlation of Carnitine levels to Methionine and Lysine intake', *Physiol Res*, vol 49, pp 399–402.

12 Laidlaw S.A. et al, 1988, 'Plasma and urine taurine levels in vegans', *Am J Clin Nutr*, vol 47, pp 660–663.

13 Schmidt J.A., 2016, 'Plasma concentrations and intakes of amino acids in male meat-eaters, fish-eaters, vegetarians and vegans: a cross-sectional analysis in the EPIC-Oxford cohort', *European Journal of Clinical Nutrition*, vol 70, pp 306–312.

14 Tang G., Qin J., Dolnikowski G. et al, 2003, 'Short-term (intestinal) and long-term (postintestinal) conversion of beta-carotene to retinol in adults as assessed by a stable-isotope reference method', *Am J Clin Nutr*, vol 78, issue 2, pp 259–266.

15 Afshin, A., 2019, 'Health effects of dietary risks in 195 countries, 1990–2017: a systematic analysis for the Global Burden of Disease Study 2017', *The Lancet*, vol 393, issue 10184, pp 1958–1972.

16 Verhoeven D.T. et al, 1996, 'Epidemiological studies on

brassica vegetables and cancer risk', *Cancer Epidemiol Biomarkers Prev*, vol 5, issue 9, pp 733–748.

17 Yu M.C., et al, 2002, 'Arylamine exposures and bladder cancer risk', *Mutation Research/Fundamental and Molecular Mechanisms of Mutagenesis*, vols 506–507, pp 21–28.

18 Kobylewski S. and Jacobson M.F., 2012, 'Toxicology of Food Dyes', *International Journal of Occupational and Environmental Health*, vol 18, issue 3, pp 220–246.

19 Oplatowska-Stachowiak M. and Elliott C.T., 2017, 'Food Colors: Existing and emerging food safety concerns', *Critical Reviews in Food Science and Nutrition*, vol 57, issue 3, pp 524–528.

20 Iyyaswamy A. and Rathinasamy S., 2012, 'Effect of chronic exposure to aspartame on oxidative stress in discrete brain regions of albino rats', *Journal of Biosciences*, vol 37, issue 4, pp 679–688.

21 Stegink L.D., Brummel M.C., Filer L.J., Baker G.L., 1983, 'Blood Methanol Concentrations in One-Year-Old Infants Administered Graded Doses of Aspartame', *The Journal of Nutrition*, vol 113, issue 8, pp 1600–1606.

22 Trocho C., Pardo R., Rafecas I. et al, 1998, 'Formaldehyde derived from dietary aspartame binds to tissue components *in vivo*', *Life Sciences*, vol 63, issue 5, pp 337–349.

23 Abhilash M., Sauganth Paul M.V., Matthews V. et al, 2011, 'Effect of long term intake of aspartame on antioxidant defence status in liver', *Food and Chemical Toxicology*, vol 49, issue 6, pp 1203–1207.

24 Pisarik P., Kai D., 2009, 'Vestibulocochlear toxicity in a pair of siblings 15 years apart secondary to aspartame: two case reports', *Cases Journal*, 2009, 2, 9237.

25 Briffa J., 2005, 'Aspartame and its effects on health', *British Medical Journal*, vol 330, issue 7486, pp 309–10.

26 Nagagawa Y., Nagasawa M., Yamada S. et al, 2009, 'Sweet taste receptor expressed in pancreatic beta-cells activates the calcium and cyclic AMP signalling systems and stimulates insulin secretion', *PLoS One*, 4 (4), e5106.

27 Pepino M.Y. et al, April 2013, 'Sucralose affects Glycemic and Hormonal Response to an Oral Glucose Load', *Diabetes Care*, DC 122221.

28 Mackenzie-Ross S.J. et al, 2010, 'Neuropsychological and psychiatric functioning in sheep farmers exposed to low levels of organophophate pesticides', *Neurotoxicology and Teratology*, vol 32, issue 4, pp 452–459.

29 Kamel F. and Hoppin J.A., 2004, 'Association of Pesticide Exposure with Neurologic Dysfunction and Disease', *Environmental Health Perspectives*, vol 112, issue 9, pp 950–958.

30 Spiewak R., 2001, 'Pesticides as a cause of occupational skin diseases in farmers', *Ann Agric Environ Med*, vol 8, pp 1–5.

31 The BSE Inquiry Report, UK Government, vol 12, section 10, statement 523, issued 23.09.1999. Patrick Holden, Director, Soil Association. Archived 25.05.2006.

32 Thomas D., 2003, 'A study on the mineral depletion of the foods available to us as a nation over the period 1940 to 1991', *Nutrition and Health*, 1st April 2003.

33 Davis D.R., 2009, 'Declining Fruit and Vegetable Nutrient Composition: What is the Evidence?', *HortScience*, vol 44, no 1, pp 15–19.

34 White P.J. and Broadly M.R., 2005, 'Historical variation in

the mineral composition of edible horticultural products', *The Journal of Horticultural Science and Biotechnology*, vol 80, issue 6, pp 660–667.

35 Lawrence, F., 2013, *Not on the Label*, Penguin Books, London.

36 Cameron E., Pauling L., 1976, 'Supplemental ascorbate in the supportive treatment of cancer: Prolongation of survival times in terminal human cancer. *Proc Natl Acad Sci USA*, vol 73, issue 10, pp 3685–89.

37 Yun J. et al, 2015, 'Vitamin C selectively kills KRAS and BRAF mutant colorectal cancer cells by targeting GAPDH', *Science*, vol 350, issue 6266, pp 1391–6.

38 Ohno S. et al, 2009, 'High-dose Vitamin C (Ascorbic Acid) Therapy in the Treatment of Patients with Advanced Cancer', *Anticancer Research*, vol 29, no 3, pp 809–815.

39 Block, G., 1991, 'Vitamin C and cancer prevention: the epidemiologic evidence', *The American Journal of Clinical Nutrition*, vol 53, issue 1, pp 270S–282S.

40 Clement, I., 1998, 'Lessons from Basic Research in Selenium and Cancer Prevention', *The Journal of Nutrition*, Volume 128, Issue 11, pp 1845–1854.

41 Clark L.C., Combs G.F., Turnbull B.W. et al, 1996, 'Effects of Selenium Supplementation for Cancer Prevention in Patients With Carcinoma of the Skin: A Randomized Controlled Trial', *JAMA*, vol 276, issue 24: pp 1957–1963.

42 Eskin B.A. et al, 1967, 'Mammary Gland Dysplasia in Iodine Deficiency: Studies in Rats'. *JAMA*. Vol 200, issue 8, pp 691–695.

43 Stadel B.V., 1976, 'Dietary Iodine and Risk of Breast, Endometrial and Ovarian Cancer', *The Lancet*, vol 307, issue 7965, pp 890–891.

44 Booth R., 6th April 2019, 'UK councils rethink use of weedkillers after US cases', *The Guardian.*

45 Kishi M., 6th June 2002, 'Initial Summary of the Main Factors contributing to incidents of acute pesticide poisoning', World Health Organisation.

46 Hurst A.F., Knott F.A., 1931, 'Intestinal Carbohydrate Dyspepsia', *QJM: An International Journal of Medicine*, vol os-24, issue 94, pp 171–179.

47 Winner H.I. and Hurley R., 1964, *Candida Albicans*, Churchill, London.

48 Truss O., 1978, 'Tissue Injury induced by Candida Albicans – mental and neurologic manifestations', *Journal of Orthomolecular Psychiatry*, vol 7, pp 17–37.

49 Truss O., 1984, 'Metabolic Abnormalities in patients with Chronic Candidiasis – The Acetaldehyde Hypothesis', *Journal of Orthomolecular Psychiatry*, vol 13, issue 2, pp 66–93.

50 Crook, W.G., 1986, *The Yeast Connection*, Professional Books, Tennessee.

51 Hunnisett A., Howard J. and Davies S., 1990, 'Gut Fermentation (or the "Auto-brewery") Syndrome: A New Clinical Test with Initial Observations and Discussion of Clinical and Biochemical Implications', *Journal of Nutritional Medicine*, vol 1, issue 1, pp 33–38.

52 Galland L. and Barrie S., 1993, 'Intestinal Dysbiosis and the causes of disease', *J Advancement Med*, vol 6, pp 67–82.

53 Eaton K.K. et al, 2001, 'A Comparison of Laculose Breath Hydrogen Measurements with Gut Fermentation Profiles in Patients with Fungal-type Dysbiosis', *Journal of Nutritional and Environmental Medicine*, vol 11, no 1, pp 33–42.

54 Eaton K.K. et al, 2002, 'Gastric Acid Production, Pancreatic Secretions and Blood Levels of Higher Alcohols in Patients with Fungal-type Dysbiosis of the Gut', *Journal of Nutritional and Environmental Medicine*, vol 12, no 2, pp 107–112.

55 Eaton K.K. et al, 2004, 'Gut Fermentation: A Reappraisal of an Old Clinical Condition with Diagnostic Tests and Management: Discussion Paper', *Journal of Nutritional and Environmental Medicine*, vol 14, no 2, pp 89–94.

56 Mosley M., 2017, *The Clever Guts Diet* (p 60), Short Books, London.

57 Fasano A., 2012, 'Leaky Gut and Autoimmune Disease', *Clinical Reviews in Allergy and Immunology*, vol 42, issue 1, pp 71–78.

58 Hollander D., 1999, 'Intestinal Permeability, leaky gut and intestinal disorders', *Current Gastroenterology Reports*, vol 1, issue 5, pp 410–416.

59 Burkitt D.P. et al, 1974, 'Dietary Fiber and Disease', *JAMA*', vol 229, pp 1068–73.

60 Ramachandran M. and Aronson J.K., 2011, 'John Bostock's first description of hayfever', *Journal of the Royal Society of Medicine*, vol 104, issue 6, pp 237–240.

61 Behrendt H. et al, 2014, 'Environmental Pollution and Allergy: Historical Aspects', *Chem Immunol Allergy*, vol 100, pp 268–277.

62 Miller C.S., 2001, 'Toxicant-induced Loss of Tolerance', *Journal of Nutritional and Environmental Medicine*, vol 11, no 3, pp 181–204.

63 Okuyama Y. et al, 2007, 'Adsorption of air pollutants on the

grain surface of Japanese cedar pollen', *Atmospheric Environment*, vol 41, issue 2, pp 253–260.

64 Gray S.L., Anderson M.L., Dublin S. et al, 2015, 'Cumulative Use of Strong Anticholinergics and Incident Dementia: A Prospective Cohort Study', *JAMA Internal Medicine*, vol 175, issue 3, pp 401–407.

65 Matta M.K. et al, 2019, 'Effect of Sunscreen Application Under Maximal Use Conditions on Plasma Concentration of Sunscreen Active Ingredients', *JAMA*, vol 321, issue 21, pp 2082–2091.

66 Calafat A.M. et al, 2008, 'Concentrations of Sunscreen Agent Benzophenone-3 in Residents of the United States: National Health and Nutrition Examination Survey 2003–2004', *Environmental Health Perspectives*, vol 116, no 7, pp 893–897.

67 Draelos Z.D., 2010, 'Are Sunscreens Safe?' (editorial), *Journal of Cosmetic Dermatology*, vol 9, issue 1.

68 Graham-Brown R. and Burns T., 2002, *Lecture Notes on Dermatology*, Blackwell, Oxford.

69 Shuster S., 21st July 2010, 'Don't let the phoney melanoma scare keep you out of the sun', *The Guardian*.

70 Berwick M. et al, 2005, 'Sun exposure and mortality from melanoma', *J Natl Cancer Inst*, vol 97, issue 3, pp 195–199.

71 Hill N. et al, 2005, 'Single blind, randomised, comparitive study of the Bug Buster kit and over the counter pediculocide treatments against head lice in the United Kingdom', *BMJ*, vol 331, pp 384–387.

72 Jägerstad M. and Skog K., 2005, 'Genotoxicity of

heat-processed foods', *Mutation Research/Fundamental and Molecular Mechanisms of Mutagenesis*, vol 574, issues 1–2, pp 156–172.

73 Trafialek J. and Kolanowski W., 2013, 'Dietary exposure to meat-related carcinogenic substances: is there a way to estimate the risk?', *International Journal of Food Sciences and Nutrition*, vol 65, issue 6, pp 774–780.

74 Mueller M.S. et al, 2004, 'Randomised controlled trial of a traditional preparation of *Artemisia annua L.* (Annual Wormwood) in the treatment of malaria', *Transactions of the Royal Society of Tropical Medicine and Hygiene*, vol 98, issue 5, pp 318–321.

75 Bendich A. and Langseth L., 1995, 'The Health effects of vitamin C supplementation: a review', *J Am Coll Nutr*, vol 14, issue 2, pp 124–136.

76 Block G., 1991, 'Epidemiologic evidence regarding vitamin C and cancer', *The American Journal of Clinical Nutrition*, vol 54, issue 6, pp 1310S–1314S.

77 Singer S.R. and Grismaijer S., 1995, *Dressed to Kill: The Link Between Breast Cancer and Bras*, Avery, New York.

78 Herr I. and Büschler M.W., 2010, 'Dietary constituents of broccoli and other cruciferous vegetables: Implications for prevention and therapy of cancer', *Cancer Treatment Reviews*, vol 36, issue 5, pp 377–383.

79 Lawrence F., 2013, *Not On The Label*, Penguin, London.

80 Chazelas E., Srour B., Desmetz E. et al, 2019, 'Sugary drink consumption and risk of cancer: results from NutriNet-Santé prospective cohort', *BMJ*, vol 366, 12408.

81 Freedman B.J., 1980, 'Sulphur dioxide in foods and beverages:

its use as a preservative and its effect on asthma', Br J Dis Chest, vol 74, issue 2, pp 128–134.

82 Zaraska, M., 2015, 'Bitter Truth', *New Scientist*, vol 227, no 3032, pp 26–29.

83 Kemp T.J. et al, 1996, 'House dust mite allergen in pillows', *BMJ*, 313:916.

84 Moss M. and Freed D., 2003, 'The cow and the coronary: epidemiology, biochemistry and immunology', *Int J Cardiol*, vol 87, issue 2–3, pp 203–216.

85 Bellingham M. and Sharpe R.M., 2013, 'Chemical Exposures During Pregnancy', *Royal College of Obstetricians and Gynaecologists*, Scientific Impact Paper no 37, May 2013.

86 Sarangi S. et al, 2010, 'Effects of exposure of parents to toxic gases in Bhopal on the offspring', *American Journal of Industrial Medicine*, vol 3, issue 8, pp 836–841.

87 Debes F. et al, 2006, 'Impact of prenatal methylmercury exposure on neurobehavioural function at age 14 years', *Neurotoxicology and Teratology*, vol 28, issue 5, pp 536–547.

88 Palmer R.F., Blanchard S., Wood R., 2009, 'Proximity to point sources of environmental mercury release as a predictor of autism prevalence', *Health & Place*, vol 15, issue 1, pp 18–24.

89 Bernard S. et al, 2001, 'Autism: a novel form of mercury poisoning', *Medical Hypotheses*, vol 56, issue 4, pp 462–471.

90 Kalter H. and Warkany J., 1957, 'Congenital malformations in inbred strains of mice induced by riboflavin-deficient, galactoflavin containing diets', *Journal of Experimental Zoology*, vol 136, issue 3.

91 Wehby G. and Murray J.C., 2010, 'Folic acid and Orofacial

Clefts: A Review of the Evidence', *Oral Dis*, vol 16, issue 1, p 11–19.

92 Smithells R.W. et al, 1980, 'Possible prevention of neural-tube defects by periconceptional vitamin supplementation', *The Lancet*, vol 315, issue 8164, pp 339–340.

93 Smithells R.W. et al, 1983, 'Further experience of vitamin supplementation for prevention of neural tube defect recurrences', *The Lancet*, vol 321, issue 8332, pp 1027–1031.

94 Laurence K.M., 1966, 'The Survival of Untreated Spina Bifida Cystica', *Developmental Medicine & Child Neurology*, vol 8, issue s11, pp 10–19.

95 Mweshi M.M. et al, 2015, 'Ethnic Pattern of Origin of Children with Spina Bifida Managed at the University Teaching Hospital and Beit Cure Hospital, Lusaka, Zambia 2001–2010', *Science Journal of Public Health*, vol 3, issue 6, pp 857–861.

96 Li Z. et al, 2006, 'A population-based case-control study of risk factors for neural tube defects in four high-prevalence areas of Shanxi province, China', *Paediatric and Perinatal Epidemiology*, vol 20, issue 1, pp 43–53.

97 Ahern M.M. et al, 2011, 'The association between mountaintop mining and birth defects among live births in central Appalachia, 1996–2003', *Environmental Research*, vol 111, issue 6, pp 838–846.

98 Favier A.E., 1992, 'The role of zinc in reproduction', *Biological Trace Element Research*, vol 32, issue 1–3, pp 363–382.

99 Keen C.L. and Hurley L.S., 1989, 'Zinc and Reproduction: Effects of Deficiency on Foetal and Postnatal Development', in Mills CF (ed) *Zinc in Human Biology*, pp 183–220.

100 Pieczynska J. and Grajeta H., 2015, 'The role of selenium in human conception and pregnancy', *Journal of Trace Elements in Medicine and Biology*, vol 29, pp 31–38.

101 Hetzel B.S., 1983, 'Iodine deficiency disorders (IDD) and their eradication', *The Lancet*, vol 322, issue 8359, pp 1126–1129.

102 Spätling L. and Spätling G., 1988, 'Magnesium supplementation in pregnancy. A double-blind study', *British Journal of Obstetrics and Gynaecology*, vol 95, pp 120–125.

103 The Magpie Trial Collaborative Group, 2002, 'Do Women with pre-eclampsia, and their babies, benefit from magnesium sulphate? The Magpie Trial: a randomised placebo-controlled trial', *The Lancet*, vol 359, issue 9321, pp 1877–1890.

104 Damien Downing, personal communication.

105 Leiser C.L. et al, 2019, 'Acute effects of air pollutants on spontaneous pregnancy loss: a case-crossover study', *Fertility and Sterility*, vol 111, issue 2, pp 341–347.

106 Lacasana M., Esplugues A., Ballester F., 2005, 'Exposure to ambient air pollution and prenatal and early childhood health effects', *European Journal of Epidemiology*, vol 20, issue 2, pp 183–199.

107 Salama A.K., Bakry N.M., Abou-Donia M.B., 1993, 'A review article on placental transfer of pesticides', *International Journal of Occupational Medicine & Toxicology*, vol 2, issue 4, pp 383–397.

108 Agarwal A. et al, 2008, 'Effect of cell phone usage on semen analysis in men attending infertility clinic: an observational study', *Fertility and Sterility*, vol 89, issue 1, pp 124–128.

109 Levine H. et al, 2017, 'Temporal trends in sperm count: a

systematic review and meta-regression analysis', *Human Reproduction Update*, vol 23, issue 6, pp 646–659.

110 Walker M., 1993, 'A fresh look at the risks of artificial feeding', *Journal of Human Lactation*, vol 9, pp 97–107.

111 Karjalainen J., Martin J.M., Knip M. et al, 1992, 'A bovine albumin peptide as a possible trigger of insulin-dependent diabetes mellitus', *New Engl J Med*, vol 327, pp 302–307.

112 Lopez-Alarcan M., Villalpando S., Fajardo A., 1997, 'Breastfeeding lowers the frequency and duration of acute respiratory infection and diarrhoea in infants under 6 months of age', *Journal of Nutrition*, vol 127, pp 436–443.

113 Silfverdal S.A. et al, 1997, 'Protective effect of breastfeeding on invasive Haemophilus influenzae infection; a case-control study in Swedish pre-school children', *Int J Epidemiol*, vol 26, pp 443–450.

114 Dagan R. and Pridan H., 1982, 'Relationship of breastfeeding versus bottle feeding with emergency room visits and hospitalization for infectious diseases', *Eur J Pediatr*, vol 139, issue 3, pp 192–194.

115 Pisacane A., Graziano L., Mazzarella G. et al, 1992, 'Breastfeeding and urinary tract infection', *Journal of Pediatrics*, vol 120, pp 87–89.

116 Duffy L.C., Faden H., Wasielewski R. et al, 1997, 'Exclusive breastfeeding protects against bacterial colonisation and daycare exposure to otitis media', *Pediatrics*, vol 100, issue 4, E7.

117 Anniansson G., Alm B., Andersson B. et al, 1994, 'A prospective cohort study on breastfeeding and otitis media in Swedish infants', *Pediatr Infect Dis J*, vol 13, pp 183–188.

118 Davis M.K., Savitz D.A. and Graubard B.I., 1988, 'Infant feeding and childhood cancer', *Lancet*, vol 2, 365–368.

119 Mitchell E.A. et al, 1991, 'Results from the first year of the New Zealand cot death study', *NZ Med J*, vol 104, pp 71–76.

120 Wright A.L. et al, 1995, 'Relationship of infant feeding to recurrent wheezing at age 6 years', *Arch Pediatr Adolesc Med*, vol 49, pp 758–763.

121 Koletzko S., Sherman P., Corey M. et al, 1989, 'Role of infant feeding practices in the development of Crohn's disease in childhood', *BMJ*, vol 298, pp 1617–1618.

122 Horwood L.J. and Fergusson D.M., 1998, 'Breastfeeding and later cognitive and academic outcomes', *Pediatrics*, vol 101, p e9.

123 Lucas A. et al, 1992, 'Breast milk and subsequent intelligence quotient in children born preterm', *Lancet*, vol 339, issue 8788, pp 261–264.

124 Andraca I. and Uauy R., 1995, 'Breastfeeding for optimal mental development' in *Behavioural and Metabolic Aspects of Breastfeeding*, ed Simopoulos A.P., Dutra de Oliveira J.E. and Desai I.D., *World Rev Nutr Diet*, Karger, Basel, vol 78, pp 1–27.

125 Taylor B. and Wadsworth J., 1984, 'Breastfeeding and child development at five years', *Dev Med Child Neurol*, vol 26, pp 73–80.

126 Newman J., 1995, 'How breastfeeding protects newborns', *Scientific American*, vol 273, pp 76–79.

127 Newcombe P.A., Storer B.E., Longnecker M.P. et al, 1994, 'Lactation and a reduced risk of premenopausal breast cancer', *NEJM*, vol 330, pp 81–87.

128 Romieu I. et al, 1996, 'Breast cancer and lactation history in Mexican women', *Am J Epidemiol*, vol 143, pp 543–552.

129 Enger S.M. et al, 1997, 'Breastfeeding history, pregnancy experience and risk of breast cancer', *Br J Cancer*, vol 76, issue 1, pp 118–123.

130 Brun J.G. et al, 1995, 'Breastfeeding, other reproductive factors and rheumatoid arthritis: a prospective study', *Br J Rheumatology*, vol 34, pp 542–546.

131 Altemus L. et al, 1995, 'Suppression of hypothalamic-pituitary-adrenal axis responses to stress in lactating women', *J Clin Endocrinol Metab*, vol 80, pp 2954–2959.

132 Tarrant R.C. et al, 2012, 'The positive role of breastfeeding on infant health during the first 6 weeks: findings from a prospective observational study based on maternal reports', *Ir Med J*, vol 105, issue 3, pp 75–78.

133 Oddy W.H. et al, 2003, 'Breastfeeding and respiratory morbidity in infancy: a birth cohort study', *Arch Dis Child*, vol 88, issue 3, pp 224–228.

134 Flores-Pajot M.C. et al, 2016, 'Childhood autism spectrum disorders and exposure to nitrogen dioxide and particulate matter air pollution: a review and meta-analysis', *Environmental Research*, vol 151, pp 763–776.

135 Grandjean P. and Landrigan P.J., 2014, 'Neurobehavioural effects of developmental toxicity', *The Lancet Neurology*, vol 13, issue 3, pp 330–338.

136 Farrow C. and Haycraft E., 2019, 'Do play with your food!', *The Psychologist*, British Psychological Society, vol 32, pp 22–25.

137 Dame Sally Davies, Chief Medical Officer, 'Antibiotic

resistance as big a threat as climate change – chief medic', *The Guardian* 29th April 2019.

138 Walton S., Wyatt E.H. and Cunliffe W.J., 1988, 'Genetic control of sebum excretion and acne – a twin study', *British Journal of Dermatology*, vol 118, issue 3, pp 393–396.

139 Blythman J., 2015, *Swallow This*, Fourth Estate, London.

140 Kranjcec B., Papes D., Altarac S., 2014, 'd-mannose powder for prophylaxis of recurrent urinary tract infections in women; a randomized clinical trial', *World Journal of Urology*, vol 32, issue 1, pp 79–84.

141 Liu G. et al, 2015, 'Nickel exposure is associated with the prevalence of type 2 diabetes in Chinese adults', *Int J Epidemiol*, vol 44, issue 1, pp 240–248.

142 Horak E. et al, 1978, 'Effects of nickel chloride and nickel carbonyl upon glucose metabolism in rats', *Ann Clin Lab Sci*, vol 8, no 6, pp 476–482.

143 Golbidi S. et al, 2011, 'Diabetes and alpha lipoic acid', *Frontiers in Pharmacology*, vol 2, p 69.

144 Packer L., Kraemer K. and Rimbach G., 2001, 'Molecular aspects of lipoic acid in the prevention of diabetes complications', *Nutrition*, vol 17, issue 10, pp 888–895.

145 Porta M., 2006, 'Persistent Organic Pollutants and the burden of Diabetes', *The Lancet*, vol 368, issue 9535, pp 558–9.

146 Scannapieco F.A., Bush R.B. and Paju S., 2003, 'Associations Between Periodontal Disease and Risk for Atherosclerosis, Cardiovascular Disease and Stroke. A Systematic Review', *Annals of Periodontology*, vol 8, issue 1, pp 38–53.

147 Damien Downing, 1988, *Day Light Robbery: The importance of sunlight to health*, Arrow Books, London.

148 Darbre P., 2016, 'Aluminium and the human breast', *Morphologie*, vol 100, issue 329, pp 65–74.

149 Gupta V.B. et al, 2005, 'Aluminium in Alzheimer's disease: are we still at a crossroad?' *Cellular and Molecular Life Sciences*, vol 62, issue 2, pp 143–158.

150 Beral V. et al, 1999, 'Use of HRT and the subsequent risk of cancer', *Journal of Epidemiology and Biostatistics*, vol 4, issue 3, pp 191–210.

151 Mahmud K., 2009, 'Natural hormone therapy for menopause', *Gynaecological Endocrinology*, vol 26, issue 2, pp 81–85.

152 Aaseth J., Boivin G. and Anderson O., 2012, 'Osteoporosis and trace elements - An overview', *Journal of Trace Elements in Medicine and Biology*, vol 26, issues 2–3, pp 149–152.

153 Hedlund L.R. and Gallagher J.C., 1989, 'Increased incidence of hip fracture in osteoporotic women treated with sodium fluoride', *Journal of Bone and Mineral Research*, vol 4, issue 2, pp 223–225.

154 Gutteridge D.H. et al, 1990, 'Spontaneous hip fractures in fluoride-treated patients: Potential causative factors', *Journal of Bone and Mineral Research*, vol 5, issue S1, pp S205–S215.

155 Sebastian A., Sellmeyer D.E., Stone K.L. et al, 2001, 'Dietary ratio of animal to vegetable protein and rate of bone loss and risk of fracture in postmenopausal women', *Am J Clin Nutr*, vol 74, issue 3, pp 411–2.

156 Heikkinen S. et al, 2015, 'Does Hair Dye Use Increase the Risk of Breast Cancer? A Population-Based Case-Control study of Finnish Women', *PLoS one*, vol 10, no 8.

157 Hamdouk M.I. et al, 2008, 'Paraphenylene diamine hair dye

poisoning', *Clinical Nephrotoxins*, pp 871–879, Springer, Boston.

158 Campbell A., 2002, 'The potential role of aluminium in Alzheimer's disease', *Nephrology Dialysis Transplantation*, vol 17, suppl 2, pp 17–20.

159 De la Monte S.M. and Wands J.R., 2008, 'Alzheimer's Disease is Type 3 Diabetes – Evidence Reviewed', *J Diabetes Sci Technol*, vol 2, issue 6, pp 1101–1113.

160 Clayton P. and Rowbotham J., 2008, 'An unsuitable and degraded diet? Part one: public health lessons from the mid-Victorian working class diet', *J R Soc Med*, vol 101, pp 282–289.

161 Smith M., Atkin A. and Cutler C., 2017, 'An Age Old Problem? Estimating the Impact of Dementia on Past Human Populations', *Journal of Ageing and Health*, vol 29, issue 1, pp 68–98.

162 Fox M., 2018, 'Evolutionary medicine perspectives on Alzheimer's Disease: Review and new directions', *Ageing Research Reviews*, vol 47, pp 140–148.

163 Grimes D.S., Hindle E. and Dyer T., 1996, 'Sunlight, cholesterol and coronary heart disease', *Q J Med*, vol 879, pp 579–589.

164 Martyn C.L. et al, 1989, 'Geographical relation between Alzheimer's disease and aluminium in drinking water', *Lancet*, vol 333, issue 8629, pp 59–62.

165 Crapper D.R., Krishnan S.S. and Quittkat S., 1976, 'Aluminium, neurofibrillary degeneration and Alzheimer's disease', *Brain: a Journal of Neurology*, vol 99, issue 1, pp 67–80.

166 Casacuberta N. et al, 2009, 'Radioactivity contents in

dicalcium phosphate and the potential radiological risk to human populations', *Journal of Hazardous Materials*, vol 170, issue 2–3, pp 814–823.

167 Schiffman S.S. and Rother K.I., 2013, 'Sucralose, a synthetic organochlorine sweetener: overview of biological issues', *J Toxicol Environ Health B Crit Rev*, vol 16, issue 7, pp 399–451.

168 Abou-Donia M.B., 2008, 'Splenda alters gut microflora and increases intestinal p-glycoprotein and cytochrome p-450 in male rats', *J Toxicol Environ Health A*, vol 71, issue 21, pp 1415–1429.

169 Dong S. et al, 2013, 'Polychlorinated dibenzo-p-dioxins and dibenzofurans formed from sucralose at high temperatures', *Scientific Reports*, 3: 2946.

170 BBC Radio 4, *The Food Programme*, Sunday 9th June 2019.

171 Hodges R.E. and Minich D.M., 2015, 'Modulation of Metabolic Detoxification Pathways Using Foods and Food-Derived Compnents: A Scientific Review with Clinical Application', *Journal of Nutrition and Metabolism*.

172 Schraufnagel D.E. et al, 2019, 'Air Pollution and Non-communicable Diseases', *Chest,* vol 155, issue 2, pp 409–416.

173 Landrigan P. et al, 2017, 'The Lancet Commission on pollution and health', *The Lancet*, vol 391, issue 10119, pp 462–512.

174 Michaelis S., 2010, 'Health and Flight Safety Implications from Exposure to Contaminated Air in Aircraft', chapter 4 of doctoral dissertation, Faculty of Science, University of New South Wales, Australia. http://www.susanmichaelis.com/phd.htm

175 Mackenzie Ross S. et al, 2011, 'Cognitive function following reported exposure to contaminated air on commercial

aircraft: methodological considerations for future researchers', *J Biol Phys Chem*, vol 11, pp 180–191.

176 Mackenzie Ross S., 2008, 'Cognitive function following exposure to contaminated air on commercial aircraft: A case series of 27 pilots seen for clinical purposes', *Journal of Nutritional and Environmental Medicine*, vol 17, issue 2, pp 111–126.

177 Schindler B.K. et al, 2013, 'Occupational exposures of air crews to tricresyl phosphate isomers and organophosphate flame retardants after fume events', *Archives of Toxicology*, vol 87, issue 4, pp 645–648.

178 Winder C. and Balouet J-C., 2002, 'The Toxicity of Commercial Jet Oils', *Environmental Research*, vol 89, issue 2, pp 146–164.

179 National Toxicology Program, 1987, 'NTP Toxicology and Carcinogenesis Studies of 1,4–Dichlorobenzene in Rats and Mice', *Natl Toxicol Program Tech Rep Ser*, vol 319 pp 1–198.

180 Passon D., 2011, 'The international crew health survey', *J Biol Phys Chem*, vol 11, pp 201–207.

181 Salmi H.A. and Sarna S., 1982, 'Effect of Silymarin on chemical, functional and morphological alterations of the liver', *Scand J Gastroenterol*, vol 17, pp 517–521.

182 Furlong C.E. et al, 2005, 'Role of paraoxonase (PON1) status in pesticide sensitivity: genetic and temporal determinants', *Neurotoxicology*, vol 26, issue 4, pp 651–659.

183 Aleynik S.I. et al, 1997, 'Polyenylphosphatidylcholine prevents carbon tetrachloride-induced lipid peroxidation while it attenuates liver fibrosis', *Journal of Hepatology*, vol 27, issue 3, pp 554–561.

184 McNeely E. et al, 2018, 'Cancer prevalence among flight attendants compared to the general population', *Environmental Health*, vol 17, issue 1, p 49.

185 Michaelis S., 2011, 'Contaminated Aircraft Cabin Air', *J Biol Phys Chem*, vol 11, issue 4, pp 132–145.

186 Winder C. and Michaelis S., 2005, 'Crew Effects from Toxic Exposures on Aircraft', in 'Air Quality in Airplane Cabins and Similar Enclosed Spaces', pp 229–248, part of *'The Handbook of Environmental Chemistry'* book series.

187 Harrison V. and Mackenzie Ross S., 2016, 'An emerging concern: Toxic fumes in airplane cabins', *Cortex*, vol 74, pp 297–302.

188 Abou-Donia M.B. et al, 2013, 'Autoantibodies to Nervous System-Specific Proteins are Elevated in Sera of Flight Crew Members: Biomarkers for Nervous System Injury', *Jnl Toxicol and Env Health*, Part A, 76: pp 363–380.

189 Thompson C.M. et al, 1988, 'Regional Brain Trace-Element Studies in Alzheimer's Disease', *NeuroToxicology*, vol 9, issue 1, pp 1–8.

190 Pendergrass J.C. et al, 1997, 'Mercury Vapor Inhalation Inhibits Binding of GTP to Tubulin in Rat Brain: Similarity to a Molecular Lesion in Alzheimer Diseased Brain', *NeuroToxicology*, vol 18, issue 2, pp 315–324.

191 Needleman H.L. et al, 1996, 'Bone lead levels and delinquent behaviour', *JAMA*, vol 275, issue 5, pp 363–369.

192 Brockel B.J. and Cory-Slechter D.A., 1998, 'Lead, attention and impulsive behaviour: changes in a fixed-ratio waiting-for-reward paradigm', *Pharmacol Biochem Behav*, vol 60, issue 2, pp 545–552.

193 Grimsrud T.K. et al, 2003, 'Lung cancer incidence among Norwegian nickel-refinery workers 1953–2000', *J Environ Monit*, vol 5, issue 2, pp 190–197.

194 Yang Y. et al, 2008, 'Urinary level of nickel and acute leukaemia in Chinese children', *Toxicol Ind Health*, vol 24, issue 9, pp 603–610.

195 Mold M. et al, 2018, 'Aluminium in brain tissue in autism', *J Trace Elem Med Biol*, vol 4, pp 76–82.

196 Darbre P.D., Mannello F. and Exley C., 2013, 'Aluminium and breast cancer: Sources of exposure, tissue measurements and mechanisms of toxicological actions on breast biology', *J Inorg Biochem*, vol 128, pp 257–261.

197 Buha A. et al, 2019, 'Bone mineral health is sensitively related to environmental cadmium exposure – experimental and human data', *Environ Res*, vol 176.

198 Djordjevic V.R. et al, 2019, 'Environmental cadmium exposure and pancreatic cancer: Evidence from case-control, animal and in vitro studies', *Environ Int*, vol 128, pp 353–361.

199 Störtebecker P., 1989, 'Mercury Poisoning from Dental Amalgam through direct Nose-Brain transport', *The Lancet*, 1: 1207.

200 Vimy M. and Lorscheider F.L., 1985, 'Clinical Science: Intra-oral Air Mercury Released from Dental Amalgam', *Journal of Dental Research*, vol 64, issue 8, pp 1072–1075.

201 Lorscheider F.L., Vimy M.J. and Summers A.O,. 1995, 'Mercury Exposure from "silver" tooth fillings: emerging evidence questions a traditional dental paradigm', *Journal of FASEB, Federation of American Societies for Experimental Biology*, vol 9, pp 504–508.

202 Nylander M., Friberg L. and Lind B., 1987, 'Mercury concentrations in the human brain and kidney in relation to exposure from dental amalgam fillings', *Swedish Dental Journal*, vol 11, issue 5, pp 179–187.

203 Uzzell B.P. and Oler J., 1986, 'Chronic low-level mercury exposure and neuropsychological functioning', *Journal of Clinical and Experimental Neuropsychology*, vol 8, issue 5, pp 581–593.

204 Mutter J. et al, 2010, 'Does Inorganic Mercury Play a Role in Alzheimer's Disease? A Systematic Review and an Integrated Molecular Mechanism', *Journal of Alzheimer's Disease*, vol 22, no 2, pp 357–374.

205 Brownstein D., 2009, *Iodine: why you need it, why you can't live without it.* Medical Alternatives Press, Michigan.

206 Bassin E.B., 2001, 'Association Between Fluoride in Drinking Water During Growth and Development and the Incidence of Osteosarcoma for Children and Adolescents', DMSc thesis, Harvard School of Dental Medicine, Boston, Massachusetts.

207 Lantz O. et al, 1987, 'Fluoride-Induced Chronic Renal Failure', *American Journal of Kidney Diseases*, vol 10, no 2, pp 136–139.

208 National Research Council, 2006, 'Fluoride in Drinking Water: A Scientific Review of EPA's Standards', chapter 7, *Neurotoxicity and Neurobehavioural Effects*, National Academies Press, Washington DC.

209 Doyle T.J. et al, 1997, 'The association of drinking water source and chlorination by-products with cancer incidence among post-menopausal women in Iowa: a prospective

cohort study', *American Journal of Public Health*, vol 87, issue 7, pp 1168–1176.

210 Bernard A. et al, 2003, 'Lung hyperpermeability and asthma prevalence in schoolchildren: unexpected associations with the attendance at indoor chlorinated swimming pools', *Occupational and Environmental Medicine*, vol 60, issue 6, pp 385–394.

211 van Leeuwen F.X.R. et al, 1983, 'Toxicity of sodium bromide in rats: Effects on endocrine system and reproduction', *Food and Chemical Toxicology*, vol 21, issue 4, pp 383–389.

212 Caldwell J., Lunn R. and Ruder A., 1995, 'Tetrachloroethylene (perc, tetra, PCE)', IARC Monographs 63.

213 Pope C.A. et al, 2002, 'Lung cancer, cardiopulmonary mortality, and long-term exposure to fine particulate air pollution', *JAMA*, vol 287, issue 9, pp 1132–1141.

214 Hayes R.B. et al, 2019, 'PM2.5 air pollution and cause-specific cardiovascular disease mortality', *Int J Epidemiol*. In press at the time of writing.

215 Calderon-Garciduenas L. et al, 2019, 'Air Pollution, Combustion and Friction Derived Nanoparticles, and Alzheimer's Disease in Urban Children and Young Adults', *J Alzheimers Dis*, vol 70, issue 2, pp 343–360.

216 Bose S. et al, 2019, 'Prenatal particulate air pollution exposure and sleep disruption in preschoolers: Window of susceptibility', *Environmental International*, vol 124, pp 329–335

217 Turner M.C. et al, 2017, 'Ambient Air Pollution and Cancer Mortality in the Cancer Prevention Study II', *Environ Health Perspect*, vol 125, issue 8.

218 Zhang Z. et al, 2018, 'Exposure to nitrogen dioxide and chronic obstructive pulmonary disease (COPD) in adults: a systematic review and meta-analysis', *Environ Sci Pollut Res Int*, vol 25, issue 15, pp 15133–15145.

219 Szyszkowicz M., Rowe B.H. and Kaplan G.G., 2009, 'Ambient sulphur dioxide exposure and emergency department visits for migraine in Vancouver, Canada', *Int J Occup Med Environ Health*, vol 22, issue 1, pp 7–12.

220 Deger L. et al, 2012, 'Active and uncontrolled asthma among children exposed to air stack emissions of sulphur dioxide from petroleum refineries in Montreal, Quebec: a cross-sectional study', *Can Respir J*, vol 19, issue 2, pp 97–102.

221 Bahadar H. et al, 2014, 'Current understandings and perspectives on non-cancer health effects of benzene: a global concern', *Toxicol Appl Pharmacol*, vol 276, issue 2, pp 83–94.

222 Bello-Medina P.C. et al, 2019, 'Ozone pollution, oxidative stress, synaptic plasticity and neurodegeneration', *Neurologia*. In press at the time of writing.

223 Greenberg M.M., 1997, 'The central nervous system and exposure to toluene: a risk characterization' *Environ Res*, vol 72, issue 1, pp 1–7.

224 Roshandel G. et al, 2012, 'Polycyclic aromatic hydrocarbons and esophageal squamous cell carcinoma', *Arch Iran Med*, vol 15, issue 11, pp 713–722.

225 Karimi P. et al, 2015, 'Polycyclic aromatic hydrocarbons and childhood asthma', *Eur J Epidemiol*, vol 30, issue 2, pp 91–101.

226 Gankhuyag N. et al, 2017, 'The role of Nitrosamine (NNK) in Breast Cancer Carcinogenesis', *J Mammary Gland Biol Neoplasia*, vol 22, issue 3, pp 159–170.

227 Peterson L.A., 2017, 'Context Matters: Contribution of Specific DNA Adducts to the Genotoxic Properties of the Tobacco-Specific Nitrosamine NNK', *Chem Res Toxicol*, vol 30, issue 1, pp 420–433.

228 Lang A.L. and Beier J.I., 2018, 'Interaction of volatile organic compounds and underlying liver disease: a new paradigm for risk', *Biol Chem*, vol 399, issue 11, pp 1237–1248.

229 Di Carlo F.J. et al, 1978, 'Assessment of the hazards of polybrominated biphenyls', *Environ Health Perspect*, vol 23, pp 351–365.

230 Infante P.F. et al, 2009, 'Vinyl chloride propellant in hair spray and angiosarcoma of the liver among hairdressers and barbers: case reports', *Int J Occup Environ Health*, vol 15, issue 1, pp 36–42.

231 Environmental Working Group, 2012, 'The Scent of Danger: Are there Toxic Ingredients in Perfumes and Colognes?' *Scientific American*, 29th Sept 2012.

232 Sonne C. et al, 2004, 'Is bone mineral composition disrupted by organochlorines in East Greenland polar bears (Ursus maritimus)?', *Environmental Health Perspectives*, vol 112, issue 17: pp 1711–1716.

233 IARC – International Agency for Research on Cancer – 'IARC Monographs vol 112: evaluation of five organophosphate insecticides and herbicides', WHO (World Health Organisation), 20th March 2015.

234 National Toxicology Program of the US Department of Health and Human Services, Report on Carcinogens, 14th edition, 1,4–Dichlorobenzene, CAS No. 106–46–7.

235 Bang du Y., Lee I.K. and Lee B.M., 2011, 'Toxicological

characterisation of phthalic acid', *Toxicol Res*, vol 27, issue 4, pp 191–203.

236 Gago-Dominguez M. et al, 2000, 'Use of permanent hair dyes and bladder-cancer risk', *International Journal of Cancer*, vol 91, issue 4: pp 575–579.

237 Waring R. and Klovrza L.V., 2000, 'Sulphur Metabolism in Autism', *Journal of Nutritional and Environmental Medicine*, vol 10, pp 25–32.

238 Ferenci P. et al, 1989, 'Randomised controlled trial of silymarin treatment in patients with cirrhosis of the liver', *J Hepatol*, vol 9, pp 105–13.

239 Anderson A., Cheng N., Bryden N.A. et al, 1997, 'Elevated Intakes of Supplemental Chromium Improve Glucose and Insulin Variables in Individuals with Type 2 Diabetes', *Diabetes*, 46(11): 1786–1791.

240 Lopez H.W., Leenhardt F., Coudray C. et al, 2002, 'Minerals and phytic acid interactions: is it a real problem for human nutrition?', *Intl Jnl Food Science & Technol*, 37(7): 727–739.

241 Coulibaly A., Kouakou B. and Chen J., 2011, 'Review Article. Phytic Acid in Cereal Grains: Healthy or Harmful Ways to Reduce Phytic Acid in Cereal Grains and Their Effects on Nutritional Quality', *American Journal of Plant Nutrition and Fertilisation Technology*, 1(1): 1–22.

242 Hotz C. and Gibson R.S., 2007, 'Traditional Food-Processing and Preparation Practices to Enhace the Bioavailability of Micronutrients in Plant-Based Diets', *The Journal of Nutrition*, 137(4): 1097–1100.

243 Freed D.L.J., 1991, 'Lectins in Food: Their Importance in Health and Disease', *Journal of Nutritional Medicine*, 2(1): 45–64.

244 Hadjivassiliou M. et al, 1996, 'Does cryptic gluten sensitivity play a part in neurological illness?' *The Lancet*, 347(8998): 369–371.

245 Whitely P. et al, 1999, 'A gluten-free diet as an intervention for autism and associated spectrum disorders: preliminary findings', *Autism*, 3(1): 45–65.

246 Mozaffarian D. et al, 2006, 'Trans Fatty Acids and Cardiovascular Disease', *NEJM*, 354: 1601–1613.

247 Boskou G. et al, 2006, 'Content of trans, trans-2,4–decadienal in deep-fried and pan-fried potatoes', *European Journal of Lipid Science and Technology*, 108(2): 109–115.

248 Bansal G. et al, 2009, 'Analysis of trans fatty acids in deep frying oil by three different approaches', *Food Chemistry*, 116(2): 535–541.

249 Chen Y. et al, 2014, 'The analysis of *trans* fatty acid profiles in deep frying palm oil and chicken fillets with an improved gas chromatography method', *Food Control*, 44: 191–197.

250 Peng C.Y. et al, 2017, 'Effects of cooking method, cooking oil and food type on aldehyde emissions in cooking oil fumes', *Journal of Hazardous Materials*, 324(B): 160–167.

251 Zahir E. et al, 2017, 'Study of physicochemical properties of edible oil and evaluation of frying oil quality by Fourier Transform-Infrared (FT-IR) Spectroscopy', *Arabian Journal of Chemistry*, 10(2): S3870–S3876.

252 Spector T., 2015, *The Diet Myth*, W&N, London.

ABOUT THE AUTHOR

Dr Jenny Goodman is a medical doctor, broadcaster and lecturer. After qualifying and working in general medicine, surgery and A&E, she did a post-graduate training in nutritional and environmental medicine that radically transformed her approach to helping patients. Jenny has been practising nutritional and environmental medicine for over twenty years, using her knowledge of human nutrition and biochemistry to investigate and treat the many and varied problems that people bring to her. Jenny is passionate about making medical and nutritional knowledge accessible to the general public and is a popular and much sought-after lecturer. She lives in north London with her husband, two adult children and a cat.

INDEX

books to help you live a good life

Join the conversation and tell
us how you live a #goodlife

🐦 @yellowkitebooks
📘 YellowKiteBooks
📌 Yellow Kite Books
📷 YellowKiteBooks